The Last Diet Book Standing

Kerry McLeod

simple nutrition series press

Gainesville, GA
www.simplenutritionseries.com

Notice:

The Last Diet Book Standing is solely for informational purposes and was designed to help you make better lifestyle choices when it comes to your health. It is not intended to replace medical advice or to be a substitute for a physician. Always consult with a medical or health professional before starting any new nutrition, weight loss, or exercise program, or if you have questions about your health in general. Neither the author nor the publisher shall be liable or responsible for any loss, injury, or damage allegedly arising from any information contained in this book.

Published by Simple Nutrition Series Press
1930 Tapawingo Drive, Gainesville, GA 30501
Orders@simplenutritionseries.com

Library of Congress Control Number: 2004092433
McLeod, Kerry

ISBN 0-9753411-0-3

Printed and bound in Colombia by Imprelibros S.A.

To my husband David and my daughter Sophie, who provide the inspiration and the motivation to be as healthy as I can be—every day.

Table of Contents

Acknowledgments

"It takes a village" is the only way to describe the team effort that has gone into making this book a reality. The "village" consists not only of a team of dedicated professionals, but also the family and friends who provided ongoing support over the past two years.

The Village People (the experts)

This book does not exist without the input, hard work, and passion that each of these experts brought to the table. There aren't enough words to describe my deepest appreciation, so I'll just say it simply—thanks to each of you from the bottom of my heart. Now, let's name names …

Gregory D. Roberts, D.D.S., M.D.—who very generously reviewed the content of the book. His feedback, based on sound medical science, was crucial in making this a healthy and complete weight loss program for women.

Natalie Logan, R.D., L.D.—our resident nutritionist who helped to organize the bulk of the nutritional content, ensuring that it flowed in an easy-to-understand format—and who basically kept me honest! She was instrumental in creating the meal plans and oversaw the tedious task of conducting the nutritional analyses on each meal.

Sara Guerin, B.S., Exercise and Sports Sciences—our resident nutrition researcher and the consummate cheerleader! She's been involved in this project from the word go. Her positive attitude, along with her excellent research skills, helped to keep this project alive and kicking over the past two years.

Jill Bennett Gaieski, Executive Editor (and best buddy since sixth grade)—her professional and invaluable contributions helped to transform my original concepts into the concrete program that exists on these pages. And, as always, she was a source of daily belly laughs that helped me through some very rocky moments with this project. We've been through all the major milestones together over the past 28 years; it just seems fitting that she would play such a large role in my most important professional accomplishment to date. She defines the word friendship. I can't wait to see what the next 28 years have in store for us!

Jeff G. Jones, Book Designer—his beautiful design and countless hours of work far exceeded even my wildest dreams of what this book could be visually. But even more than that—the dedication and friendship that he displayed throughout this VERY long and never-ending process will not be forgotten. I am glad to call him my friend!

Pat Fraser, Copy Editor (and new friend)—talk about a true professional and one of the easiest people in the world to work with. She expertly guided the manuscript through the final editing stages, but more than that, she made the hideous process (for me, anyway) of editing and correcting every last word not only tolerable but enjoyable too!

John Guerin, great brother and friend, and phenomenal artist—he's the brainchild behind the title of the book and the boxing-glove theme. He not only set up the entire photo shoot so that all I had to do was show up and smile (and wear the boxing gloves), but also provided the encouragement and confidence I needed to go out on this emotional limb. A special thanks to the ladies at the Hill Country Bookstore in Georgetown, Texas, for allowing us to use their store for the photo shoot!

Mindy Carter, Cover Designer (and new friend)—an extremely talented designer who "gets it" right off the bat. She's a pleasure to work with on all levels and a girl who's cut from the same cloth!

The Village People (the family)

I must thank my always supportive, always hilarious, and sometimes crazy family. First and foremost to my mom, who still teaches me life lessons every day; to my father, who even at this late date is still showing me that with hard work and determination any goal can be achieved; to my sisters, Jen and Sue, the two best friends a girl could have—and who always let me know when I'm being the village idiot; to my brothers, Bob and John—the two funniest people alive—who have always taken care of me; and to my nieces, Sara and Gaby, who are so sweet and beautiful, and are in charge of keeping me "in the know" with the latest fashions! A special thanks to Carol, the best mother-in-law in the world—she's truly a godsend to our family. And last, but not least, to my husband David, who really picked up the slack at home so I could finally finish this book—thanks for sticking with me until the bitter end!

Mom

A Note About Mom, Our Mascot

Women today are extremely busy. Whether it be with our own activities or taking care of others, we tend to put our own nutrition and health needs on the back burner. Let's face it, most of us could use a friendly reminder to eat right, to exercise, and to make better lifestyle choices—and who better to remind us than Mom?

Throughout this book you will see little notes from—you guessed it, Mom. Her messages are well intentioned and offer sage advice. They can be sarcastic and even make you feel guilty at times—and usually rightfully so. But—they will always leave you smiling! She's the mom you didn't always listen to when you were younger, but once you got older (and wiser), wish that you had. So here's **your chance** to do it all over again, except this time do it right, and listen to her. After all, aren't moms usually right?

With that, I'd like to make a special dedication to my mom—Fran. She's the best! It's truly the only way to describe her. It took having a husband, a child, and turning forty for me to realize that she's usually right about most things. I no longer make a move without her input—it's like having a built-in "life consultant" who thankfully doesn't charge by the hour!

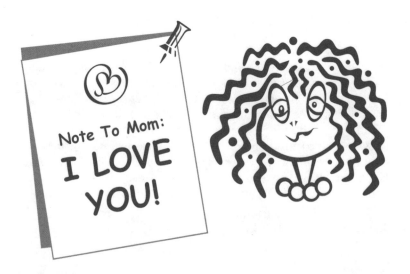

Note To Mom:
I LOVE YOU!

Introduction

Something Is Amiss In The Weight Loss World

There are thousands of diet and nutrition books on the market today. Yet, Americans are more overweight and unhealthy than ever. The conclusion: There's something amiss in the weight loss world. But don't despair—we've gotten to the bottom of it!

After reviewing some of the most popular nutrition books, the top diet programs, and the latest and greatest fitness and health magazines, here's what we found: an abundance of very sound, valuable, and useful information in every form and fashion that clearly conveys what we should do to be healthier and thinner. And here's what we didn't find: a one-stop resource that not only told us what to do, but showed us how to do it every step of the way!

We were looking for a weight loss and nutrition program that didn't exist. We wanted a plan that would take us by the hand and make the process simple. That would explain the most important information in a fun and easy-to-read format. That would show us how to personalize a plan for our individual lifestyles. That would show us exactly what to buy at the grocery store, down to the last detail. That would provide the tools for creating, implementing, and tracking a new eating plan—for life. And, most important, one that would provide a central headquarters for everything we need—when we need it. So, to fill the void in the weight loss world, we took these key elements and used them as the blueprint to create this book, and more specifically, our turnkey eating plan that we call Simple Nutrition For Life.

And now you know why this will be The Last Diet Book Standing on your bookshelf—it's the total package for all your weight loss and nutrition needs!

Okay, enough about us—back to you. Read on to find out what this program includes, what it doesn't include, what's in it for you, the steps to implement it, and how long it will take for you to see results.

What Is The Simple Nutrition For Life Plan?

The **Simple Nutrition For Life** plan is a one-stop resource that includes everything you need to manage your nutritional and weight loss goals for life! It will help you stay focused and organized, and achieve the three B's—**A Better Body, Better Health, and a Better Life!**

It's designed in a step-by-step format to help you create a personalized eating plan based on **YOUR** lifestyle. It includes a set of realistic, healthy lifestyle guidelines, easy-to-access reference materials, and a variety of meal selections. Plus, essential planning and activity sheets designed in a "day timer" format to help you stay organized and on track with your new lifestyle goals. But here's the best part—this nutrition and weight loss companion comes in a portable format you can take anywhere! So, when you need it, it's there.

We've told you what the program includes. Now we think it's important to clarify what the program doesn't include so that we can set realistic expectations for you. Our program will not provide:

◄ **A short-term diet that gives you instant but temporary results.**

◄ **A major detailed explanation about the 40 nutrients that the body needs and how they work.**

◄ **Instructions on eliminating certain food groups that provide quick weight loss** (i.e., carbs or fat)**.**

◄ **Appetite suppressants or "fat burning" supplements to help "kick start" your weight loss plan.**

If you are in the market for an eating plan that includes any of these, this program is not for you! You may as well close the book and use it as a doorstop. Even though our program is simple, it **DOES** require you to look at your current lifestyle habits, make some smart and easy changes, and adhere to some basic nutritional guidelines.

What Makes Our Concept Unique?

The **Simple Nutrition For Life** concept is simple. It's permanent weight loss through healthy lifestyle habits, better nutrition, and portion control. Nothing new about this concept. It's tried and true and proven to work. However, what is unique about our program is the means to the end—the way we help you achieve your goals. We call it The Simple Nutrition Planning System.

The Simple Nutrition Planning System is the "total package" when it comes to weight loss and good nutrition, because it includes five key elements that are designed to give you the power to finally create a personalized eating plan that will help you feel and look great! Take a look.

The unique features of our program by section include:

1. Simple Nutrition 101

We believe that information is power, but we also think that too much information can be overload. So we opted for a happy medium that doesn't bog you down with a lot of detail and jargon that in the long run are more confusing than helpful. Rather, we provide you with just the stuff you need to make better lifestyle choices by combining the most important rules of nutrition and weight loss in an easy-to-read format.

2. Multi-Task Meals and More

Our meal plan stays true to its name by helping you to multi-task at every meal. Our meals are packed with nutrition and great taste, and are easy to prepare—even if you're on the go! Designed by professionals, they're packed with disease-fighting foods, anti-aging benefits, and guaranteed to satisfy your hunger and cravings! To make things super easy we created the Ultimate Shopping List that includes our top 21 most nutritious foods, plus we scoured grocery store shelves to come up with our list of best brands by food group. We've taken the guesswork out of healthy meal planning by providing everything you need on a silver platter!

3. Personal Makeover Plan Worksheets

We've designed one-of-a-kind worksheets that will help you to easily and quickly create a realistic eating and weight loss plan based on your lifestyle and your goals. We have found that if you have a hand in creating your own action plan, and it really fits your lifestyle, you will be more likely to stick with it and ultimately reach your goals!

4. The Simple Nutrition Organizer

We've also developed one-of-a-kind activity sheets in a "day timer" format that will help you to stay organized while executing your plan. This section includes weekly meal planning sheets (we even have a place for daily "to-do's"), weekly grocery list sheets, and a journal for daily progress reports. It's one thing to have a great plan, but quite another to put it into action and see it through. With these activity sheets, you can't miss.

5. The Ultimate Cheat Sheets

We've created easy-to-reference "cheat sheets" that provide important stuff you'll need every day—like rules on reading food labels, healthy substitutes for your favorite foods, and tips on portion control. We don't expect you to remember everything; we just want you to know where to find it when you need it!

What's In It For Me?

Okay, here's the "what's in it for you" part. If you follow our program consistently, you can count on these things:

◁   **A personalized eating plan that will help you maintain your weight for life!**

◁   **Increased confidence about being healthier and achieving your goal weight.**

◁   **Enjoying tasty meals that are easy to prepare, and pack a nutritional punch.**

◁   **A planning system to help organize all your nutrition needs.**

◁   **Increased awareness of how nutrition helps to lower your risk of chronic diseases.**

◁   **Finding the secret to prolonging the aging process, from the inside out.**

◁   **More energy than you've had in years!**

In a nutshell, our program gives you the most important rules of nutrition and weight loss with a no-fail planning, organizing, and tracking system that takes you from **A-Z** in **YOUR** quest for the ultimate eating plan. The final result: **A Better Body, Better Health, and a Better Life.** Can you ask for more than that?

When Can I Expect To See Results?

Good question. The answer is, it's up to you. First, it depends on how much you need to clean up your lifestyle and eating habits. Second, it depends on your commitment to making these changes and sticking to them. For instance, if losing weight is your main goal, our plan will show you how to lose one to two pounds per week—safely and effectively—by using the 8-week nutrition and meal planner, which is designed to help you create and tweak an eating plan that is just right for you.

Remember, this isn't a crash or fad diet; it's a plan for life. By trading high-fat, empty-calorie meals for meals packed with nutrition, you'll immediately feel better and have more energy. Stick to it and your weight will be where you want it for life! So, if you are ready to create your very own **"Simple Nutrition For Life"** eating plan, then let's begin.

First, we want to share with you The 7 Habits of Highly Healthy Women—these lifestyle habits are key to succeeding with our plan! ▶

The 7 Habits of Highly Healthy Women

> **Things we'll cover in this chapter:**

- ▶ **How to achieve the three B's**
- ▶ **Easy transition to healthy habits**
- ▶ **The payoff**
- ▶ **The 7 healthy lifestyle habits**

Following a healthy lifestyle is not that difficult—IN THEORY. Sure, it boils down to a few basic guidelines that are simple and logical. They include things like: eating a balanced diet, watching our portions, and exercising often. Sounds simple enough, yet so many of us are doing just the opposite. Why? Frankly, we have gotten ourselves into a rut of unhealthy habits! Our lives are more hectic than ever, so we look for convenience. Between work, school, socializing, hobbies, and the kids, there's no time to eat right or to exercise—and we're paying the price with our health.

Can You Get Out Of Your Unhealthy Lifestyle Rut?

Yes, and it won't be hard, **BUT** it will involve a commitment to making some changes in your current lifestyle—there's no getting around this. Therefore, you have to be ready, really ready, to make the necessary changes—this is the key to succeeding with this program. And you're obviously on the road to being ready because you're reading this book, which is the first step towards **A Better Body, Better Health, and a Better Life!**

Tips For Making Changes

Remember, healthy lifestyle habits are really pretty simple; it's just a matter of knowing what they are and how to easily incorporate them into your everyday life. Before we give you the 411 on the healthy habits, here are a few pointers that will help you make the transition from unhealthy to healthy habits less traumatic:

◄ **Focus on making new, "healthy" habits, rather than focusing on breaking bad habits; psychologically, it will be easier.**

◄ **Don't reinvent the wheel; the beauty of the Simple Nutrition For Life program is that we give you all the information you need to make better choices, along with the necessary tools. All you have to do is implement the program!**

◄ **Instead of stressing out over an all-or-nothing approach, think in terms of moderation. We don't promote complete abstinence from junk food, mainly because it's unrealistic, it's too inflexible, and frankly, it's no fun! Instead, we promote moderation and making better lifestyle choices.**

Note from Mom:
If you're reading this book with a soda in one hand and a candy bar in the other, maybe you're not quite ready to make changes at this time, and that's okay. Because when you are, I'll be here for you. I'm an optimist; I believe there's always tomorrow, Scarlet!

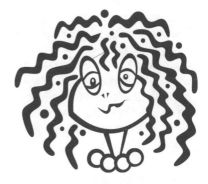

What's The Payoff?

The payoff for incorporating healthy habits into your lifestyle can be tremendous and well worth the effort. Just making a few small changes in your overall eating plan and moderately exercising most days can help lower your risk of many chronic diseases. Not to mention, prolong the aging process, help you to lose unwanted pounds, and maintain a healthy weight permanently! For instance, making a small change like cutting out 100 calories a day (a small soda or that extra cookie) would result in a 10-pound weight loss over a period of one year. Imagine if you added a few more healthy food choices, portion control, and consistent exercise to the mix! —There would be no living with you!

So let's begin by example. The following are what we determined to be the "lifestyle habits" of **Highly Healthy Women.** Make a mental note of how many of these are habits you are already hooked on.

The 7 Habits Of Highly Healthy Women

Habit #1: Highly Healthy Women make health, nutrition, and weight management a priority.

No matter how busy you are, the most important thing is your health. The key to good health is taking preventive measures every day, like eating right and exercising consistently. These measures will help you maintain a healthy weight—plus they'll help ward off chronic diseases, which is so important. Equally important is early detection of diseases through regular health screenings appropriate for your age group. And on a superficial note, being at a healthy weight will make you feel great, will give you more confidence, and will make everything you do more enjoyable!

Habit # 2: Highly Healthy Women have a game plan for success that includes planning and tracking their meals.

They plan out meals in advance.

Daily and weekly menu planning is the key to staying on course with your nutritional and weight loss goals. Prepare a shopping list before you go to the store and try to stick to buying only those items. Remember, if you stock your fridge with healthy foods, you're probably going to eat them. Also, prepare meals and snacks in advance; it makes it less likely that you will grab something unhealthy when you are hungry.

They keep a food and exercise diary.

It's a fact: people who write down what they eat are twice as likely to eat healthier, lose weight, and keep it off. Most diet/nutrition experts agree that recording your meals and snacks keeps you honest. You'll be amazed at how many calories you didn't realize you were consuming—this will help to avoid a very serious condition —**Calorie Amnesia!**

Habit #3: Highly Healthy Women make wise food choices every day.

Being healthy and maintaining your goal weight is not just a matter of eating less, it's also about making better food choices that still provide great taste and pack a nutritional punch. The easiest way to do this is to include the healthiest selections from the five food groups, with an emphasis on getting your 5 to 10 fruits and veggies and enough fiber each day! By doing this, you will retrain your mind and body to go for more whole foods (health protective), rather than unhealthy, fatty, processed, packaged junk foods. After a few days of cutting out the "bad stuff" and substituting it with the "good stuff," your body will begin to crave the "good stuff"—we guarantee it!

Habit #4: Highly Healthy Women eat 5 to 6 mini-meals per day.

There are several ways to safely speed up your metabolism. Exercise is one way and eating more often is another. Smaller meals help you ward off hunger and avoid overeating. When you get too hungry because you've skipped meals, it puts the body into starvation mode, signaling your metabolism to slow down. Then when you finally do feed your body, you run the risk of binge eating. So eating often is the best way to increase your metabolism.

They eat breakfast.

Breakfast literally kick-starts your day and your metabolism! By eating that first meal, you give yourself calories (read: energy) to get going. Studies show that most adults are more productive after a well-balanced breakfast. If time is an issue, grab a food that travels well and eat it in the car, on the train, or at your desk once you get to work.

Habit #5: Highly Healthy Women practice safe portion control.

Adhering to the recommended serving sizes from the major food groups automatically keeps your calorie count in check. Restaurants and fast-food places serve portions that are 2 to 5 times larger than they were in the 1950's—no wonder we are fatter! By consistently eating smaller portions of food, you'll begin to be satisfied with these portions; it only takes a few days for the body to adjust.

Habit #6: Highly Healthy Women drink 8 cups of water per day.

Staying hydrated helps rid your body of toxins, reduces stress levels, enhances your metabolism, and makes you feel fuller. Try to limit your intake of alcohol and caffeine, as they tend to be dehydrating. **Tip:** don't leave home without a water bottle. You can get a lot of water drinking done in the car, while waiting at appointments, when shopping, and of course, while exercising. **PS: Don't forget your portable snacks too.**

Habit #7: Highly Healthy Women exercise consistently.

Exercise is one way to speed up your metabolism (remember, eating frequent small meals is another). Both cardio and strength training are very effective in maintaining weight long term because they burn calories while building muscle. At rest, each pound of muscle burns about 35 calories a day, while a pound of fat burns only two calories. **You do the math!**

Exercise can also make your bones stronger, it beats stress, fights off mild depression, and can help you sleep better at night.

These healthy habits seem basic, right? However, trying to incorporate them all into your daily life at one time might be hard to digest. And that's where we come in. With the **Simple Nutrition For Life** plan, we'll show you how to get your nutritional and weight loss house in order by providing a step-by-step format to help you create your very own personal eating and lifestyle plan. After all, it's **your life**, so it should be **your plan**.

Okay, Let's Review:

◄ Due to our hectic lives, convenience eating, supersized fast food, and sedentary ways, many of us are in an unhealthy rut.

◄ Being "mentally ready" is key in succesfully incorporating new, healthy habits into your lifestyle.

◄ Moderation is the name of the game. Eating healthy most of the time leaves less room for the unhealthy stuff.

◄ The big payoff for incorporating healthy habits into your life can be A Better Body Better Health, and a Better Life!

Note to self: Sounds sort of easy. I'm going to give this a try so I can be a Highly Healthy Woman too.

In Section 1, Simple Nutrition 101, you'll learn the basic rules of nutrition and weight loss, and why they are so important to your health—and your waistline. ▶

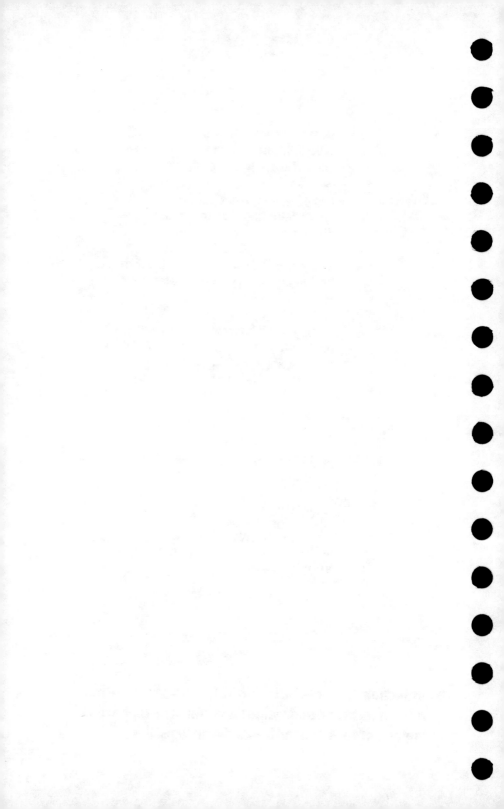

Section 1

Simple Nutrition 101 ▶

Chapter 1

When Bad Foods Happen to Good People

Things we'll cover in this chapter:	▶ The typical American diet
	▶ The bad effects of a poor diet
	▶ The positive effects of a good diet
	▶ Foods contributing to chronic diseases

Did you know that our nation is more overweight and unhealthier than ever? And that the percentage of many diseases that are plaguing Americans has skyrocketed over the past 20 years? One out of every four deaths in this country today is from cancer.

So what is causing us to be so overweight and unhealthy? Experts say that it's a combination of genetics, the environment, and the American lifestyle—mainly the diet.

Well, there's not much we can do about our genetics—we are who we are. In terms of the environment, we can do our part to help make the world a safer place to live, but so much of it is out of our control. And then there's our diet. This is the one thing we can control. — There's some food for thought.

Portrait Of An Unhealthy Diet

Let's take a minute to review the typical American diet. Overall, our diets consist of highly processed, packaged convenience-type foods. They are loaded with artificial colors and flavors and chock-full of bad fats. On the next page is a closer look.

Most Americans' diets are:

- Deficient in fruits and vegetables and other plant-based foods.
- Too low in fiber and too high in refined (processed) grains.
- Too high in saturated fats from animal foods.
- Too high in trans fats from fast-food meals and packaged goods.
- Too high in sodium and refined sugar from commercially baked goods.

What's Wrong With This Diet?

For starters, there are almost no whole foods in this diet. By "whole foods," we mean fruits, veggies, legumes, nuts, and whole grains. Instead, it's basically made up of too much fat, too little fiber, and a bunch of man-made, processed ingredients that are hard to pronounce. This type of diet over a long period, combined with lack of exercise, has been proven to contribute to the onset of many chronic diseases. _These unhealthy foods actually help to lower the immune system's ability to ward off chronic diseases_—and they make us fat to boot!

Bad Food Fallout

Each and every day we hear new scientific evidence that ties poor nutrition to the onset of chronic diseases, and that a healthier diet can actually help ward off illness. Take a look at the effects a poor diet can have:

- Over 60% of Americans are overweight/obese.
- 35% of all cancers are related to diet.
- Obesity has increased by 40% in adolescents in the past 20 years.
- 60% of the deaths in America due to heart disease and stroke are diet related.
- At least 16 million people in the U.S. have pre-diabetes—where diet is a major factor.
- More than 20 million Americans are affected by osteoporosis; studies show that it can be diminished through diet.
- The annual economic impact of these chronic diseases in the U.S. exceeds 200 billion dollars—and that affects us all!

Amazing Effects Of A Healthy Diet

The Simple Nutrition For Life view that alterations in the diet that include healthier choices can positively impact your health is backed by sound medical data. But don't take our word for it; read on.

◄ **Healthy food habits can help you reduce three of the major risk factors for heart attack—high blood cholesterol, high blood pressure and excess body weight, as well as reduce your risk of stroke.** (American Heart Association)

◄ **A diet high in fruits and vegetables can help prevent cancer over a lifetime.** (American Cancer Society)

◄ **Consuming a healthy diet is one of the best ways to prevent or combat heart disease.** (Harvard Nurses' Health Study)

◄ **Nutrition and physical activity can help ward off Type II diabetes.** (American Diabetes Association)

◄ **Some ways in which osteoporosis can be prevented include a proper diet, weight-bearing exercises, limited alcohol intake, and not smoking.** (College of American Pathologists)

◄ **High levels of antioxidants and zinc found in fruits and vegetables significantly reduce the risk of advanced age-related macular degeneration and its associated vision loss.** (Archives of Ophthalmology)

Why Are "Good People" Still Eating "Bad Foods"?

We live in an age of convenience, where fast food and instant gratification are glamorized through the overload of junk food marketing. Technology has made us sedentary, increased work schedules have made the desire for "convenient foods" irresistible and our food portions have become supersized. These things, coupled with the fact that consumers are confused by misleading and conflicting nutritional information, are making the American public sick to death, literally. — We're in a pickle, as they say.

On the next page, we list the leading food categories that are contributing to the high rate of chronic diseases in our society. Do a mental check to see how many of these foods you eat in a single week, or worse, in a single day. If your diet consists of most of these foods, you just might be nutritionally bankrupt!

Full-fat meats: are high in saturated fats and calories, and some are high in nitrates. **Examples include:** prime rib, bacon, deli meats, hot dogs, and regular ground beef.

Full-fat dairy products: are high in saturated fats and calories. **Examples include:** "whole" milk, yogurt, cheese, cream cheese, and ice cream.

Unhealthy oils: are hydrogenated and contain trans fats. **Examples include:** lard, palm oil, coconut oil, margarine, and vegetable shortening.

Fast foods: are high in saturated fats, trans fats, and calories. **Examples** (like you need any) **include:** double cheeseburgers, burgers with sauces and high-fat dressings, hot dogs, French fries, and onion rings.

Commercially baked goods: are high in processed white flour, trans fats, and refined sugars. **Examples include:** donuts, pastries, pies, and cakes.

Packaged snacks: many of them are made with partially hydrogenated oils (trans fats), olestra, artificial additives, high sodium, and refined sugars. **Examples include:** potato chips, crackers, cookies, and breakfast foods (i.e., cereals, breakfast bars, and toaster pastries).

Sugary beverages: contain artificial dyes, refined sugar, and corn syrup. **Examples include:** sodas, punches, and fruit drinks.

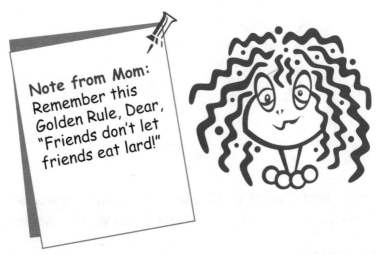

Note from Mom:
Remember this
Golden Rule, Dear,
"Friends don't let
friends eat lard!"

Okay, Let's Review:

◄ Too many Americans are making poor diet choices.

◄ Poor nutrition is a major factor in chronic diseases and deaths.

◄ A healthy diet can help to lower the risk of many chronic diseases and actually help save lives.

◄ Diet is the one thing that each individual has control over.

Note to self:
Making an effort to improve my diet by making better food choices is kind of a no-brainer.

In the next chapter, you'll learn what a healthy diet looks like and how to easily incorporate it into your hectic life.

Portrait of a Healthy Diet

You learned in the last chapter that an unhealthy diet plays a major role in being overweight and in the onset of many chronic diseases, and that a healthy diet could be your best defense. Doesn't it make sense that you should try to eat a healthier diet? The answer is a big fat yes!

Now, in order to incorporate a healthy eating plan into your already hectic life, you should first understand what a healthy eating plan looks like and what makes it healthy in the first place. In other words, we think you need to understand the basics of nutrition before you will have success with the Simple Nutrition For Life plan.

Healthy Eating 101

We believe a healthy eating plan is based on simply consuming a variety of foods each day so you get the nutrients needed for good health. Here's what a healthy eating plan looks like:

◀ **It's high in fruits and vegetables.**
◀ **It's high in plant-based foods** (legumes).
◀ **It's high in whole grains** (fiber).
◀ **It includes low-fat dairy and low-fat meat selections** (low in saturated fats).
◀ **It's low in fast-food meals.**
◀ **It's low in processed snacks and desserts** (low in trans fats, sugar, and sodium).

This eating plan is healthy because it consists mainly of "whole foods" like whole grains, fruits and veggies. It's also low in saturated fats, and it's low in processed foods—which means it's automatically lower in trans fats, refined sugar, and sodium. We stress these smart choices along with portion control because together they can produce permanent weight loss, and can help prevent chronic diseases.

Just The Basics Please

It is important to understand on a basic level that, in order to function properly, your body requires a certain amount of energy and nutrients from carbohydrates, protein, fats, water, vitamins, and minerals every day. Additionally, you should have enough fiber, calcium, and plenty of antioxidants and phytochemicals each day to achieve maximum health. Because no one food provides all the nutrients that your body needs, eating a wide variety of foods ensures that you get the necessary nutrients that promote good health.

But Don't Take Our Word For It: According to the National Academy of Sciences' Institute of Medicine, you should follow these daily dietary guideline ranges:

Carbohydrates ▸ **45-65% of total calories** (includes grains, fruits, and veggies)

Protein ▸ **10-35% of total calories** (includes dairy, meat, legumes, and soy)

Fat ▸ **20-30% of total calories** (10% or less from saturated & trans fats)

Calcium ▸ **1,000-1,200 mg** (women over 50 need 1,200 mg per day)

Fiber ▸ **21-25 grams** (women over 50 only need 21 grams per day)

Sodium ▸ **2,400 mg or less**

Cholesterol ▸ **300 mg or less**

Sugar (added) ▸ **40 grams or less**

Water ▸ **8 cups or more**

Okay, all this is fine and good, but now you need to know how to easily incorporate this into your everyday life.

The simplest way to meet these guidelines and to get all the nutrients you need each day is to use the Food Guide Pyramid as a general guide. It's not meant to be a rigid prescription but simply a guide that lets you choose a healthy diet that's right for you.

Food Guide Pyramid
A Guide to Daily Food Choices

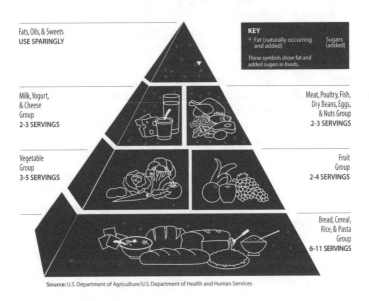

KEY
○ Fat (naturally occurring and added)   Sugars (added)

These symbols show fat and added sugars in foods.

Fats, Oils, & Sweets
USE SPARINGLY

Milk, Yogurt, & Cheese Group
2-3 SERVINGS

Meat, Poultry, Fish, Dry Beans, Eggs, & Nuts Group
2-3 SERVINGS

Vegetable Group
3-5 SERVINGS

Fruit Group
2-4 SERVINGS

Bread, Cereal, Rice, & Pasta Group
6-11 SERVINGS

Source: U.S. Department of Agriculture/U.S. Department of Health and Human Services

This guide suggests getting the majority of your daily calories from plant foods like bread, cereal, rice, pasta, fruits, and vegetables, while eating animal foods like meat, poultry, fish, and eggs less often, and of course, eating processed sweets and fats sparingly.

Note: We think it's important to clarify that fats, oils, and sweets are not considered a "food group" but they do occur naturally in many foods. For instance, salmon and avocados are great sources of good fat. In addition, you will find natural sugars that are accompanied by antioxidants, phytochemicals, and fiber in fruit. These types of fats and sugars are essential to good health. It's the processed foods that contain added trans fats and added sugars that should be consumed sparingly.

The Food Guide Pyramid's Dirty Little Secret

While this guide does a good job of distinguishing the best food groups, it fails to distinguish between the healthiest and unhealthiest foods within each food group. For example, all grains are not created equal! There's a big difference between whole grains and refined grains. It also fails to mention that low fat or skim milk is a healthier choice than whole milk. But don't despair! The **Simple Nutrition For Life** plan provides the best selections within each group so YOU don't have to think about it.

The Pyramid also suggests daily serving ranges from each of the major food groups (see diagram on the previous page). The number of servings right for you depends on how many calories you need in a given day to maintain a healthy weight. Sounds sort of complicated, don't you think? And that's where we come in. In Section 3, we'll show you how to create your own personal calorie budget, along with the appropriate servings from each food group, based on your specific needs. Keep in mind, though, almost everyone should have at least the lowest number of servings in the ranges for each food group.

It is also very important to know what the standard serving sizes (portions) are for the various foods found in the Food Guide Pyramid. Incorporating portion control into your eating plan will be the key to weight management. This concept is so important to the success of the **Simple Nutrition For Life** plan that we dedicated a whole chapter to it (Portion Distortion, Chapter 5).

The Major Food Groups

Here's the inside scoop on the major food groups. To make things really simple, we also list the healthiest as well as the unhealthiest food choices for each food group on page 34. Make a mental note of how many of the foods you eat on a regular basis from the "best choices" list. If it's not many, you may be a perfect candidate for a **Nutrition Makeover!**

The Grain Group

The grains, also known as carbohydrates, are the body's fuel of choice and should make up the largest percentage of your daily calories. However, these days they seem to have a "bad rap" for making us fat, which couldn't be further from the truth. It's the type of grains you choose that makes a difference—whole grains trump refined grains every time. Plus, it's **how much** you eat of a certain food that matters when it comes to weight gain. Whole grains are essential for good health. They contain B vitamins, iron, zinc, folic acid, and minerals, and are packed with phytochemicals; they are naturally low in fat, and provide slow, constant energy. In addition, they're a great source of fiber, which flushes out toxins and keeps your digestive system running smoothly. Fiber can be a dieter's best friend because it fills you up, has no calories, and packs a huge nutritional punch. Combined, these things help to lower blood cholesterol, assist the body with absorbing fewer calories, and help reduce the risk of many cancers, heart disease, diabetes, and strokes. —**Why would anyone want to eliminate these from their diet?**

Compare this to the fact that refined grains are processed foods, which automatically means they are less nutritious, and they are often higher in calories. For instance, refined flours made from wheat have about **66%** of the B vitamins removed, **70%** of the minerals removed and **79%** of the fiber removed. Although manufacturers fortify these processed grain products with vitamins, you're still losing most of the important fiber, antioxidants, and minerals.

The bottom line on the grain group is that whole grains should be the mainstay of any eating plan, while refined, processed grains should be avoided whenever possible.

But Don't Take Our Word For It: The American Dietetic Association has condemned high-protein/low-carb diets as being dangerous because eating a diet high in fat at the expense of severely restricting protective whole grains, and nutrient-rich fruits and vegetables is not a healthy practice. The health problems associated with these diets are they increase the risk of heart disease, certain cancers, osteoporosis, and kidney disease. Lastly, because these diets cannot usually be maintained long term, people tend to revert to their old eating habits, thus gaining most of their weight back and sometimes more.

▶

The Fruit/Veggie Group

Also carbohydrates, fruits and vegetables are loaded with fiber, many essential vitamins and minerals, and are packed with phytochemicals, which may be our most potent weapon against disease. Plus, they are low in calories and fat, so they help you maintain your weight, and are natural anti-aging sources that help to maintain healthy skin, hair, and nails. They pack a nutritional punch to say the least!

Variety is the spice of life and key when it comes to this food group because each fruit and veggie brings a different set of nutrients to the table.

Tip: The deeper the color the better!

In most cases, raw fruits and veggies are the best way to go (we recommend that you wash them well). However, frozen is a close second and sometimes just as nutritious as the fresh because most are picked fully ripe and then frozen immediately, preserving the original nutritional makeup. Canned is fine too, but watch for added salt and sugar.

The Meat & Alternatives Group

This group consists of meat, poultry, fish, beans, eggs, soy, and nuts. It's also known as the protein group and contains essential nutrients for healthy muscle mass, skin, hair, eyes, and nails.

Animal selections (meat, fish, and poultry) provide a great source of B vitamins, iron, zinc, and protein. Plant-based selections (beans, soy, and nuts) are an excellent alternative to meats because they provide a great source of fiber and protein, they are naturally low in fat and calories, and are packed with phytochemicals.

Tip: Remember to drain and rinse canned beans to remove some of the added sodium.

It's important to note that not all dietary proteins are created equal. The emphasis should be on the fish and the plant-based proteins because there is considerable evidence that these foods can reduce the risk of developing heart disease. Red meat is fine in moderation, but stick to the leanest selections you can find—for instance, filets and loin cuts are good and tasty choices.

The Dairy & Alternatives Group

Milk and dairy products are an excellent source of protein, calcium, and vitamin D—making them a triple whammy on the nutrition front. Great alternatives to the dairy group are enriched soy products.

These foods help to strengthen and promote healthy bones and teeth, and are instrumental in helping to prevent osteoporosis and in slowing the aging process. New research shows that they even help the body burn excess fat!

Much like the meat group, it is important to know that when choosing dairy products, the whole-fat choices are full of saturated fats, which can outweigh many of the benefits you might receive. Make a conscious effort to choose low fat or nonfat dairy selections.

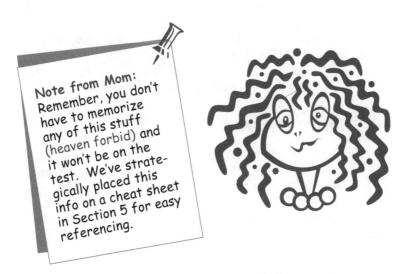

Note from Mom:
Remember, you don't have to memorize any of this stuff (heaven forbid) and it won't be on the test. We've strategically placed this info on a cheat sheet in Section 5 for easy referencing.

Best Food Selections From The Food Groups

Since no single food provides all the nutrients that the body needs, eating a wide variety of foods ensures that you get the nutrients necessary to promote good health! Below are some of the healthiest food choices within each food group. See how many of these you can fit into your new eating plan!

Grains

Whole-grain breads, whole-grains (brown rice, long grain, basmati, quinoa), whole-wheat tortillas, whole-wheat pastas, oatmeal (slow cooking) and high-fiber cereals.

Fruits and veggies

Mango, papaya, kiwi, apricots, bananas, pineapples, citrus fruits, melons, red grapes, berries, dark green leafy veggies (spinach, romaine lettuce, and broccoli), dark yellow veggies (carrots and sweet potatoes), tomatoes, red peppers, mushrooms, and garlic.

Meat & Alternatives

Lean beef (round, loin, sirloin, shank, flank, chuck, and filet), lean pork (tenderloin, center loin, and ham), veal (all cuts except ground), lamb (leg, loin, and fore shanks), skinless poultry, fish and shellfish, whole eggs or egg whites, raw nuts and seeds, all natural peanut butter, legumes (beans and peas), soy products (soybeans, edamame, soy nut butter, tofu, and tempeh).

Dairy & Alternatives

Skim milk or low-fat milk, "reduced-fat" cheeses, cottage cheese, yogurt, cream cheese, sour cream, frozen yogurt or ice cream, enriched light soymilk, and soy cheese.

Worst Food Selections From The Food Groups

Below are some of the most <u>unhealthy</u> food choices by food group. Although we don't promote complete abstinence from these foods, we do suggest you try to limit them to no more than 10% of your overall daily diet!

Grains

White bread, white rice, white pasta, most muffins, pastries, donuts, and sugary cereals.

Fruits and Veggies

Veggies that are overcooked or boiled, canned in heavy syrups or high sodium, high-fat foods that contain fruits (ice cream or yogurt), and fruit drinks that are high in calories and sugar.

Meat & Alternatives

Full-fat meats (bacon, sausage, prime rib, and hot dogs), cured luncheon meats, and poultry with skin.

Dairy & Alternatives

"Whole-fat" milk, yogurt, cottage cheese, cream cheese, sour cream, cheese, and ice cream.

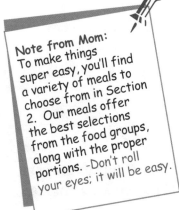

Note from Mom:
To make things super easy, you'll find a variety of meals to choose from in Section 2. Our meals offer the best selections from the food groups, along with the proper portions. -Don't roll your eyes; it will be easy.

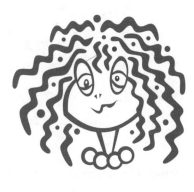

Okay, Let's Review:

◀ A healthy diet consisting of whole foods that are low in saturated fats and minimally processed can help prevent the onset of many diseases.

◀ Following the recommended number of daily servings from each food group, along with portion control, will help with long-term weight management.

◀ The simplest way to get good nutrition is to choose the best selections from the major food groups.

◀ The major food groups supply more than 40 important essential nutrients.

Note to self:
In order to keep my bottom in line, I should eat a well-balanced diet and watch my portions. Eating a healthy diet could be my best defense against many diseases. I gotta try this!

In the next chapter, you'll see why healthy fats are essential to weight management and in preventing diseases.

Chapter 3

The Skinny on Fat

Things we'll cover in this chapter:

- ▸ **Good fats vs. bad fats**
- ▸ **Trans fats and how to avoid them**
- ▸ **The truth behind "low-fat" packaged foods**

Because there is so much controversy about "fat" and the role it plays in weight management and our overall health, we thought it warranted its own chapter. Consider this the "everything you ever wanted to know about fat, but were afraid to ask" section.

First, it's important to know that not all fats are created equal. There's good fat, bad fat, nonfat, low fat, full fat, and the list goes on. Second, you learned in the last chapter that fats/oils should be used sparingly; however, they are absolutely an essential part of good health and maintaining your weight. So that you can easily identify the healthy fats from the unhealthy fats, we've divided them into three categories for your reading pleasure. They are **the good, the bad, and the ugly.**

Before we get started, there are two interesting **fat facts** you should know:

- ◂ A nonfat diet can actually cause you to gain weight! How can that be? Well, it's scientifically proven that the body stores what is in short supply for as long as possible. So, if you deny your body fat, it is going to hold onto what fat you already have. —I hate when that happens.

- ◂ All fats have more than twice the calories (9 calories per gram) of carbs and protein (each has 4 calories per gram). So, good or bad, it is important to watch your fat intake.

The Good Fats

The good fats (unsaturated) can actually help you lose weight because they help the body burn fat rather than store it. They also help to lower **LDL** cholesterol levels (bad cholesterol) and maintain or even raise **HDL** (good cholesterol). It's important to include good fats at every meal, because they help to absorb other nutrients like vitamins A, D, E, and K more efficiently. The recommended amount of good fats should be in the range of 20-30% of your total daily calories. There are two types of good fats:

Monosaturated fats are <u>usually</u> liquid at room temperature, but can start to solidify in the refrigerator. The main sources include olives, olive oil, canola oil, peanut oil, most nuts, and avocados.

Polyunsaturated fats are <u>usually</u> liquid at room temperature and in the fridge. Main sources include vegetable oils such as safflower, corn, sunflower, soy and cottonseed. Another type of polyunsaturated fat, called omega-3 fatty acids, are well known to provide a wide range of health benefits. They appear to decrease the risk of heart attacks, protect against irregular heartbeats, and lower blood pressure levels. In addition, they may protect against some cancers. They are found mainly in fish, such as salmon, mackerel, and herring. Lesser amounts are found in flaxseeds, walnuts, soybeans, and canola oil.

The Bad Fats

The bad fats (saturated) contribute to arterial aging and heart disease, as well as strokes and many different types of cancer and diabetes, because they raise bad cholesterol and suppress the good. They are solid at room temperature and are found most often in animal products such as red meat, poultry, butter, eggs, and whole milk products like ice cream, cheese, and cream cheese. Other foods high in saturated fats include coconuts, coconut milk, coconut oil, and palm oil. It is important to note that many of the saturated fat-ladden products, like butter, mayo, cream cheese, and salad dressing, are offered in low fat or nonfat versions, which are far better choices. The recommended daily amount of saturated fat is <u>10% or less</u> of your total calories.

The Ugly Fats

The ugly fats (trans fats) along with saturated fats are thought to raise your blood cholesterol levels and increase your risk of heart disease, Type II diabetes, and other serious health problems. Trans fats are made when hydrogen is added to vegetable oil through a process called hydrogenation; this makes the fat more solid at room temperature. It helps to increase the shelf life of foods, and supposedly makes them taste better. Often, trans fats are found alongside saturated fats in products such as vegetable shortening, margarine, crackers, cookies, candy, commercially baked goods, and fried/processed foods.

But Don't Take Our Word For It: Trans fats are all the rage in the media right now for two reasons. First, the FDA recently took the position that "intake of trans fats should be as low as possible," but refused to set a maximum recommended daily allowance because they stated the only <u>safe level is zero.</u> Second, food manufacturers are not presently required to list the amount of trans fats in their products. So, many seemingly "heart-healthy" foods, made with vegetable oils containing little saturated fat and no cholesterol, do contain this very "heart-unhealthy" trans fat.

<u>Good news!</u> The FDA has mandated that the food manufacturers list the amount of trans fats found in their products. They have until January 2006 to include this on the Nutrition Facts label. Some large food companies have already started to implement the new labeling and several others have begun taking steps to reduce and/or eliminate trans fats from their products. —**Three cheers for the Red, White, and Blue!**

Hydro What?

In the meantime, if you see the words **hydrogenated** or **partially hydrogenated** in the ingredients listed on food labels, you should know the food contains trans fats. That's your cue to try to avoid eating that particular food. However, you will find that it's quite a challenge to avoid buying packaged foods that don't have trans fats in them. Look at the foods you purchase each week, even the ones that you thought were super healthy. You'll be amazed at how many of them contain trans fats. Don't get discouraged! Check out our list of packaged foods **that don't** contain trans fats on our Best Brands List in Section 4.

▶

Chewing The Fat On "Low Fat"

Finally, let's talk about the "low-fat" this and "nonfat" that scam. Here's a rule of thumb: If it sounds too good to be true, it usually is. Apply this theory to most low-fat packaged foods. Here's why. The low-fat versions of packaged food (cookies, cakes, crackers, etc.) may sound like healthier alternatives to the regular versions. But, truth be told, manufacturers often compensate for the lack of fat by adding more sugar, salt, and thickeners to boost flavor and texture, thereby substituting one evil for several others. And here's the real kicker. Low-fat versions usually have about the same number of calories (sometimes more) as the regular versions.

If you compare the labels, you'll find "low-fat" is not the same as "low-calorie." In addition, you'll quickly realize that because most low-fat versions don't taste as good, you tend to eat more to satisfy that craving. You're probably better off eating the full-fat cookie that you were craving in the first place, but limit one per customer please.

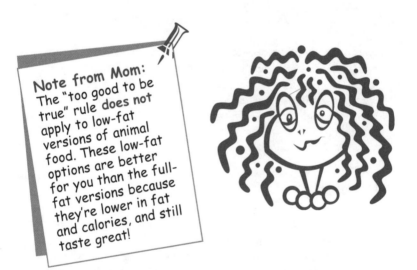

Note from Mom:
The "too good to be true" rule does not apply to low-fat versions of animal food. These low-fat options are better for you than the full-fat versions because they're lower in fat and calories, and still taste great!

Okay, Let's Review:

◄ Make sure to include foods high in the essential fatty acids for optimum health. However, you only need a little bit of even the good stuff to get the protective benefit; any more will make you fat.

◄ When using fat as a spread, choose the lower-fat versions (i.e., low-fat salad dressings, mayo, butter, and cream cheese).

◄ "Low-fat" animal foods are great options and still taste great. However, low-fat package goods often contain other unhealthy ingredients, lack taste, and are not typically lower in calories.

◄ Keep consumption of saturated and trans fats to a minimum. They can make you fat and are linked to major diseases.

Note to self:
When fat is good, it's very, very good. When fat is bad, it's very, very bad. But, too much fat, good or bad, can make me fat!

In the next chapter, you'll learn some great tips on how to read food labels in order to make the healthiest food choices at the grocery store. ▶

Chapter 4

A Crash Course in Label Reading

Things we'll cover in this chapter:

- ▶ Reading between the lines on food labels
- ▶ Finding hidden fats, sugars, sodium, and more
- ▶ Things to look for on Nutrition Facts labels

This is an important chapter because knowing what to look for on a label can make or break your nutrition and weight loss bank. Unfortunately, you cannot always rely on food manufacturers to have your best interest at heart (pardon the pun). They seem to go out of their way to emphasize "healthy" ingredients when mostly they've added miniscule amounts. And, often, there are other unhealthy ingredients —like trans fats—in their products that outweigh the good stuff. As an unsuspecting shopper, you may think you're making a wise food choice, but in reality, these products have little nutritional value. — **Don't you feel cheated?**

There are three areas on a packaged food item that you should get familiar with to keep your body healthy and slim. They include the "front label," the "ingredients list," and the "Nutrition Facts" label. Manufacturers use the front label to entice shoppers to buy their products—it's pure advertising. The ingredients list actually tells you most of what's in the food item. The Nutrition Facts label tells you how nutritious the food item is by showing how much of each nutrient a serving contains. Taken together, the information on all three labels will help you make the healthiest food choices.

How To Avoid Being Tricked By Food Labels

We recommend that you speed read through the front label of food packages because there are no mandated rules that manufacturers must follow. In other words, they can imply that a food item is very nutritious even if it's not. However, the ingredients list and the Nutrition Facts label can give you the clues you need to figure out whether a food item is a wise choice. Below is just one example of a product where the front label would indicate a healthy choice. But take a closer look; you will see that this food is nutritionally bankrupt on so many levels. Just as an FYI, we've changed the brand name to protect the guilty!

Exibit A: Yummy Fruit & Grain Yogurt Bars

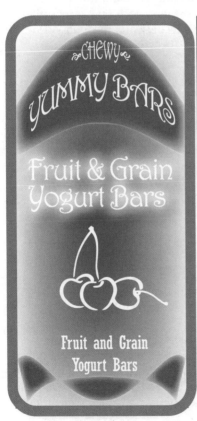

Nutrition Facts

| Serving Size | 1bar(37g) |
| Servings per Package | 8 |

Amount/Serving	
Calories	140
Fat Calories	25

	% Daily Value*
Total Fat 3g	5%
Unsaturated Fat 0.5g	3%
Cholesterol 0mg	0%
Sodium 110mg	5%
Total Carbohydrates 27g	9%
Dietary Fiber 1g	4%
Sugar 14g	
Protein 2g	

Calories Per gram: Fat 9 - Carbohydrates 4 - Protein 4

Ingredients: Filing (high fructose corn syrup, glycerin, water, fructose, modified corn starch, partially hydrogenated cottonseed and soybean oil,nonfat yogurt powder[yougurt is heat-treated after culturing], blueberries, modified tapioca starch, malic acid, corn starch, natural and artifical flavor, salt, color added, cellulose gum, carmel color, soy lecthi, red #40), enriched whole flour, whole oats, sugar, partially hydrogenated soybean and/or cottenseed oil, high fructose, corn syrup, honey, calcium carbonate, dextrose, non fat dry milk, wheat bran, salt, cellulose gum, leavening (potassium bicarbonate), natural and artifical vanilla flavor, soy lecithin, wheat gluten, corn starch, niacinamide, carrageenan, guar gum, zinc oxide, reduced iron, pyridoxine hydrochloride, riboflavin, Vitamin A and folic acid.

The front label implies a nutritional snack that is packed with fruit, grains, and yogurt—sounds very healthy and tasty!

However, when you look at the actual ingredients list and the Nutrition Facts label, this is what you will find:

- ◄ **Partially hydrogenated cottonseed and soybean oil** (code for trans fat)
- ◄ **Artificial fruits**
- ◄ **Nonfat yogurt powder** (contains no active cultures)
- ◄ **Added refined sugars** (enough said)
- ◄ **Only one gram of fiber** (code for the "grain" is largely white flour)

The manufacturer does enrich the product with calcium and vitamins. But an enriched food is code for processed, which means the healthy stuff has been removed in the manufacturing "process." In other words, the good nutrients have been removed along with the fiber and other vitamins and minerals, so the manufacturer has to further process to artificially add some nutrients back into the food. —Does that even make sense?

Now you see that only when you read the entire product label can you make a wise food choice. Would you agree this is not really a healthy choice? So, as a wanna-be nutrition-savvy shopper, you need to begin reading between all the lines!

More About Label Trickery

Here are some other front label tricks to watch out for:

"Fortified," "enriched," "added," "extra," and "plus": these words usually mean the food has been altered or processed in some way.

"Fruit drinks": these words usually mean little to no fruit and a lot of sugar. Instead, look for products that say "100% fruit juice."

"Made with wheat," or "rye," or "multi-grains": these words imply it's a good source of whole grains. Unfortunately, manufacturers are not legally required to say how much whole grain is in the product on the front label. Look for the word "whole" before the grain on the ingredients list to ensure that you are actually getting a whole-grain product.

"Natural" or "made from natural": these words simply mean the manu-facturer <u>started</u> with a natural source. Once processed, the food may not resemble anything "natural."

"Organically grown," "organic," "pesticide-free," and "no artificial ingredients": these words say very little about the nutritional value or safety of the product. Trust only those labels that say "certified organically grown."

"Sugar-free," "sugarless," or "no added sugar": these words may be misleading, because products using these terms may contain sugar alcohols, a derivative of sugar, which yield as many calories as table sugar (4 calories per gram).

The Proof Is In The Pudding

The ingredients list label will help you find the hidden saturated and trans fats, sugars, sodium, artificial flavorings, and refined grains. Ingre-dients are listed in order of most to least amounts. That means the first ingredient will be in the largest quantity. The second is the second most and so on. For instance, if a product claims to be a "fruit breakfast bar," look for fruit to be one of the top two ingredients. If you see "enriched wheat flour" or "sugar" before the fruit, put it back on the shelf and make a better choice!

In addition to the bad ingredients discussed above, try to avoid foods that contain these "evildoer" ingredients whenever possible:

- ◄ **Olestra:** a fake fat that eliminates good vitamins from your system and can cause major digestive upset—how yummy!

- ◄ **"Enriched flour," "wheat flour," or "unbleached wheat flour":** code for refined flour with just a small amount of whole wheat added.

- ◄ **"Partially hydrogenated" or "hydrogenated oils":** code for trans fats.

- ◄ **Nitrates:** used to preserve meats and have been linked to creating a powerful cancer-causing chemical in the body; found especially in luncheon meats.

▶

- **High fructose corn syrup:** a fancy phrase for refined sugar. Other forms of sugar to watch out for in the ingredients list include: honey, molasses, fruit juice concentrate, evaporated cane juice, malt, dextrose and, of course, sugar.

- **Lard shortening:** pure animal fat, enough said!

- **Artificial colorings:** chemicals used to add color to foods.

- **Monosodium glutamate** (MSG): a form of sodium; other words that mean high sodium include brine, disodium phosphate, garlic salt, onion salt, sodium alginate, sodium benzoate, sodium caseinate, sodium hydroxide, sodium nitrate, sodium pectinate, sodium propionate, sodium sulfite, baking powder, baking soda, and soy sauce.

There are more ingredients that we could list, but in the interest of saving space, here's a rule of thumb: if a food item is packed with lots of ingredients that you can't pronounce, you should look for a better food choice. Try to stick with products that are made from whole foods, with few preservatives, with few artificial sounding ingredients, and definitely no trans fats.

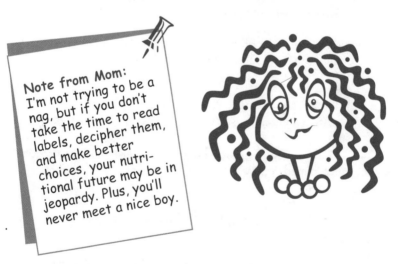

Note from Mom:
I'm not trying to be a nag, but if you don't take the time to read labels, decipher them, and make better choices, your nutritional future may be in jeopardy. Plus, you'll never meet a nice boy.

The Nutrition Facts label tells you the calories, total fat, saturated fat, cholesterol, sodium, total carbs, and protein <u>in one serving from the food item</u>. Always check the number of servings per container, listed at the top of the food label. If you eat the whole package, multiply all of the nutritional information—including the calories—by this number.

Below are a few more tips about the information on the Nutrition Facts label:

Fiber: If a product claims to be "high fiber" it should have at least 5 grams of fiber.

Reminder: Recommended daily intake of fiber is 25 grams for women under the age of 50 and 21 grams for women over the age of 50.

Sodium: If a product is low in sodium it will have less than 140 mg per serving. If it has over 400 mg, it is very high in sodium and you should try to avoid this food item, or at least watch your sodium intake for the rest of the day. It is important to note that most of the sodium you eat is added during food processing, yet another reason to stay away from processed foods! Be especially cautious of the sodium content in canned products, many boxed or frozen meals, and processed meats (bacon, sausage, and ham).

Reminder: Recommended daily intake of Sodium is 2,400 milligrams or less.

Sugar: This substance is trickier than the rest, because the Nutrition Facts label does not distinguish between added sugar and natural sugar. The distinction is very important to your health and weight loss goals, because sugar that occurs naturally in a food generally comes packaged with vitamins, minerals, and fiber, or all three. Added sugar contributes calories but no nutrients—so try to avoid foods that contain a lot of it. For instance, sodas, cereals, baked goods, breads, condiments, canned fruits in heavy syrup, fruit drinks, jams, and some alcoholic beverages are usually packed with added sugar.

Here's a rule of thumb: Be sure to read the ingredients label to see if there is any sugar added (refer to the list of code words for sugar on the previous page). When no form of sugar is listed, all the sugar is natural to the food. For instance, you'll see relatively high sugar values on labels of those foods made with milk, fruit, fruit juice, and some vegetables, but it's natural sugar. A cup of plain yogurt contains 16 grams of sugar; that's fine because it's all natural sugar. A cup of flavored yogurt might contain 33 grams of sugar because it's been sweetened; in this case, 17 grams of sugar have been added, half of your daily recommended added sugar allotment.

Reminder: Recommended daily "added sugar" should be less than 40 grams a day.

Okay, Let's Review:

◄ **You simply cannot believe everything you read! The front labels are used to sell and entice shoppers and they can be misleading.**

◄ **The ingredients label will help you find the hidden saturated and trans fats, sugars, sodium, artificial flavorings, and refined grains.**

◄ **If you can't pronounce an ingredient** (and it sounds artificial), **it's probably not a healthy choice.**

◄ **The Nutrition Facts label tells you the calories, total fat, cholesterol, sodium, total carbs, and protein** <u>in one serving from the food item</u>. **Always check the number of servings per container.**

Note to self:
I have to take responsibility for my own nutritional health and welfare when it comes to choosing food items off the grocery store shelves!!

In the next chapter, you will learn that portion control is key in maintaining your weight long term.

Chapter 5

Portion Distortion

Things we'll cover in this chapter:	▸ Standard serving sizes of foods
	▸ Eyeballing a standard serving size
	▸ Tips for keeping portions in check

So far, you've learned that good nutrition is vital to good health. Now it's important to understand that portion control is vital to weight management. Even if you eat only healthy foods, if the portions are too large (read: you take in more calories than you burn), you will probably still gain weight. The secret to good health and weight management is making wise food choices while consuming appropriate portions.

Are Your Portions Supersized?

Over the past three decades, portion sizes have increased two- to five fold in the United States. We are so used to monstrous servings that we often forget what a standard portion size really is. The number of overweight kids has more than doubled over the last 30 years (according to the Centers for Disease Control) because larger portion sizes have become the norm. Check this out: in the 1950's, the average fast food order of fries was about 2 oz; today it's two to three times larger. A hamburger was 1 oz; today it's 4 –10 oz. The average soft drink was about 7 oz; today it's 12 oz or more.

The popularity of these supersized servings means one thing—many Americans are suffering from a disorder we like to call Portion Distortion. Are you one of them?

What Exactly Is Portion Distortion?

Portion Distortion is just that. You think you are eating reasonable portions at mealtime. In fact, you actually think you are doing quite well in the diet and nutrition department. And then, low and behold, your jeans are skintight. So you think to yourself: "Something's amiss, maybe the dry cleaners have shrunk my clothes—**AGAIN**. I ate so many healthy foods. Why is this happening?"

Does this sound familiar? If so, you may be a **Portion Distortion** sufferer. Take the following short quiz to find out.

<u>**Question:**</u> Do you think the bagel you ate at the local bagel shop is 1 serving from the grain group?

<u>**Answer:**</u> No! The average bagel shop bagel is about 4 servings from the grain group and 400 calories (not to mention the cream cheese, chopped liver, and other divine toppings).

<u>**Reality check:**</u> Half of a small bagel is 1 serving from the grain group; it's the size of ½ of a hockey puck and contains about 80 calories. An entire small bagel would be 2 servings and 160 calories.

<u>**Question:**</u> Do you think a pint of orange juice is 1 serving of fruit?

<u>**Answer:**</u> No. It's actually 4 servings and over 400 calories.

<u>**Reality check:**</u> A true serving of OJ is about 6 oz, the size of a small juice glass, and has about 90 calories.

Question: Do you think a full bowl or plate of pasta is 1 serving from the grain group?

Answer: No. It's probably closer to 4 servings and over 400 calories (not including the sauce or any other added goodies).

Reality check: A true serving of cooked pasta is ½ cup, the size of a cupped hand, and contains about 100 calories. (with no sauce).

Question: Do you think the steak that you ordered from your favorite steak place is 1 serving from the meat group?

Answer: No. It's probably at least 3 servings and contains about 500 calories.

 Reality check: A serving of beef from the meat group is about 3 oz, the size of your palm, and contains about 165 calories.

If you answered "yes" to any of these questions, then you are indeed a Portion Distortion sufferer, and you may have just solved the mystery behind your behind!

Stamp Out Portion Distortion

The best way to put an end to this dreaded condition is to understand what the "standard" portions are by food group, and retrain yourself to adhere to the "standard" serving sizes. Learn to say "no" to the super-sized portions that have become the norm. You will reduce your calorie intake, and you will not feel deprived, especially if you follow the recommended daily number of servings per food group.

A serving is not just the amount you put on your plate—it's a specific amount of food defined in measurements such as cups, ounces, and pieces. It's a real eye opener to see what really constitutes a "normal" serving size, as seen on the quiz on page 50. It's important to be able to eyeball standard serving sizes, because like most people, you probably don't carry around a food scale in your purse. **Call me crazy.**

Learning to recognize and control portion sizes is a major step in eating a healthy diet and maintaining your weight long term. This way, when you happen to overdo it at a particular meal, it's okay because now you know how to compensate by eating less at your next meal or increasing your physical activity. It's not an all-or-nothing proposition!

> **But Don't Take Our Word For It:** A recent flurry of scientific research on U.S. portion sizes has transformed two previously unconfirmed beliefs into hard scientific facts: U.S. portion sizes have never been bigger, and bigger portions encourage overeating by as much as 56 percent. Source: American Institute for Cancer Research (AICR)

Talk To The Hand!

The best way to eyeball a "standard" serving size by food group is to use your trusty hand—more handy than carrying around a food scale! Your palm, fingers, and fist are the appropriate sizes for measuring ideal portions. Use the guide below to eyeball standard serving sizes.

Food	Standard Size	Eyeball
Rice /pasta	½ cup cooked	Handful (cupped)
Dry cereal	½ cup	Handful (cupped)
Fruit/veggie	½ cup	Handful (cupped)
Leafy greens	1 cup	2 cupped hands
Meat	3 oz	Your palm (size and thickness)
Milk/yogurt	1 cup	Your fist
Cheese	1 oz	Your thumb (length and width)

Other Tips For Keeping Portions In Check

In addition to eyeballing portion sizes, here are some other tips to avoid overdoing it.

◄ **When dining out, eat half of your entrée and take the other half home to be used as another meal** (remember, most restaurants serve portions that are way over the standard serving sizes).

◄ **Avoid upsizing meals and beverages at restaurants, fast food places, movie theaters, and convenience stores.**

◄ **Use smaller plates when dining at home, and don't feel obligated to clear your plate.**

◄ **Buy single serving packages of snack foods because they provide ready-made portions for you.** (Remember to read labels and buy the healthier brands!)

◄ **Munch on whole pieces of fruit that come packaged in their own natural serving sizes** (i.e., bananas, apples, and oranges).

◄ **When eating at home or dining out, think in terms of "ones." In other words, just put one scoop of food on your plate; i.e., one piece of meat; one piece of bread; one scoop of mashed potatoes. If you're still hungry, fill up with steamed veggies or salad.**

◄ **Avoid digging into a bag of potato chips or carton of ice cream. Put a portion into a bowl, and eat it. Put the rest of the food away!**

In Section 5, we have a cheat sheet dedicated to standard serving sizes for some of the best food selections per food group. We show you how to eyeball them, plus give the calorie counts. ▶

Okay, Let's Review:

◄ Over the past 30 years, portion sizes have increased two-to fivefold in the U.S.

◄ Americans have unconsciously made supersized portions the norm.

◄ The number of overweight kids has more than doubled over the last 30 years because of larger portion sizes.

◄ The "standard serving size" is a specific amount of food defined in measurements such as cups, ounces, and pieces.

◄ Eyeballing the "standard" portion sizes by food group can be done by utilizing your hand. Use your palm, fingers, and fist for figuring ideal portions.

Note to self:
Now that I know what a real serving size is, I am going to make an effort to watch my portions so that I can get back into my jeans!

In the next chapter, you'll see firsthand that making better food choices when planning your meals can shave calories while boosting nutrition!

Chapter 6

Nutrition Makeovers

Things we'll cover in this chapter:

▶ Simple ways to make healthier food choices
▶ Examples of some popular meal "makeovers"
▶ The payoff for making better food choices

After learning the difference between a poor diet and a healthy diet, you are probably beginning to realize that your current eating plan is in serious need of a **nutrition makeover.** In this chapter, we will show you how making just a few simple food selection changes can make a huge difference in the nutrients and calories that you consume.

As we keep saying, it's all about making better choices! Chances are, the meals that you're already eating can easily be made healthier and with fewer calories by simple substitution and controlling portion sizes. The payoff, guaranteed, is losing unwanted pounds and maintaining a healthy weight permanently! You may even increase your life expectancy, prolong the aging process, and help prevent many life-threatening diseases.

Here's what we've done. We've taken several of the most common meals for breakfast, lunch, and dinner, and have given them a total makeover! Our makeover meals trade empty calories for calories packed with fiber, vitamins, minerals, phytochemicals, and antioxidants. Additionally, our meals are lower in calories because we pare down the portion sizes. After reviewing these makeovers, we hope you will see that you can still enjoy your favorite meals while becoming healthier and slimmer.

Simple Nutrition Makeovers

Before ➤ **After**

Cereal & Milk
1 cup of Whole Grain Cheerios
1/2 cup of 2% milk
1 banana
Calories: 290 Fat: 7g

Cereal & Milk
1 cup of Fiber One
1/2 cup of skim milk
1 banana
Calories: 270 Fat: 2g

The payoff:

◄ Substituting the Cheerios with the Fiber One cereal provides 11 grams of additional fiber!

◄ Substituting 2% milk with skim milk, reduces fat by 4 grams.

◄ This makeover packs a huge nutritional punch with the extra fiber, fewer fats, and less calories.

Before ➤ **After**

Bagel & Juice
1 large plain bagel
1 T cream cheese
8 oz glass of orange juice
Calories: 520 Fat: 8g

Bagel & Juice
1 small whole-wheat bagel
1 T nonfat cream cheese
4 oz glass of orange juice
Calories: 260 Fat: 2g

The payoff:

◄ Substituting the large bagel with a small bagel saves about 180 calories, and switching to whole wheat provides 2 extra grams of fiber.

◄ Substituting the whole-fat cream cheese with nonfat reduces fat by 4 grams.

◄ Substituting the large glass of OJ with a smaller glass of OJ provides 55 fewer calories.

◄ This makeover saves 260 calories by adhering to standard serving sizes. Plus, you're getting more fiber and less fat.

Before ➤ After

Turkey Sandwich
6 oz of turkey breast
1 hoagie roll
1 T of mayo
½ of a pickle
1 oz of potato chips
12 oz can of soda
Calories: 750 Fat: 20

Turkey Sandwich
3 oz of turkey breast
1 whole-wheat pita (6")
1 T of Dijon mustard
1 cup of spinach leaves
2 tomato slices
1 oz of blue corn chips
Calories: 460 Fat: 12

The payoff:

◄ Reducing the portion size of the turkey to 3 oz adheres to the standard serving size for the meat group and saves 140 calories.

◄ Substituting the hoagie roll with the whole-wheat pita adds 2 grams of fiber.

◄ Substituting the mayo with mustard eliminates 5 grams of fat.

◄ Adding the extra spinach and tomatoes provides 2 servings of vegetables.

◄ Substituting the potato chips with the blue corn chips eliminates 3 grams of fat and all the trans fats.

◄ Substituting the soda with water saves 150 calories along with the refined sugar and additives.

◄ This makeover saves about 290 calories, adds 2 servings of vegetables, and eliminates 8 grams of fat!

Before ➜ **After**

Grilled Chicken Salad
3 oz of grilled chicken
2 cups of iceberg lettuce
1 diced tomato
2 oz of cheddar cheese
2 T of ranch dressing

Calories: 560 Fat: 39

Grilled Chicken Salad
3 oz of grilled chicken
2 cups of fresh spinach
2 diced tomatoes
1 oz of feta cheese
¼ cup of shredded carrots
1 T of vinaigrette
Calories: 350 Fat: 15

The payoff:

◀ Substituting the iceberg lettuce with fresh spinach provides a huge antioxidant boost, plus adding the carrots and the additional tomato provides 2 extra servings of veggies.

◀ Substituting the cheddar cheese with a smaller portion of feta cheese saves 135 calories and reduces fat by 13 grams.

◀ Substituting the full-fat ranch dressing with the smaller portion of vinaigrette saves 75 calories and reduces fat by 11 grams.

◀ This makeover saves about 210 calories, reduces fat by 24 grams, and provides 2 additional servings of veggies that are packed with antioxidants and phytochemicals.

Before ➜ **After**

Spaghetti with Meat Sauce
2 cups of pasta
2 cups of meat sauce
(Made with regular ground beef)
2 T of Parmesan cheese
12 oz can of soda
Calories: 880 Fat: 23

Spaghetti with Meat Sauce
1 cup of whole-wheat pasta
1 cup of meat sauce
(Made with very lean ground beef)
1 T of Parmesan cheese

Calories: 345 Fat: 13

The payoff:

◄ Substituting the refined white flour pasta with whole-wheat pasta and adhering to the standard portion size saves 220 calories and adds 4 grams of fiber.

◄ Using lean ground beef reduces fat by 8 grams.

◄ Adhering to the standard serving size of meat sauce saves 165 calories.

◄ Substituting the soda with water saves 150 calories.

◄ This makeover saves 535 calories, mainly by adhering to standard serving sizes. It also reduces fat by 10 grams and includes 4 extra grams of fiber.

Before ➡️ After

Meat and Potatoes	Meat and Potatoes
6 oz Rib Eye	3 oz of pork tenderloin
1 medium baked potato	1 medium sweet potato
1 T of butter	2T of low fat sour cream
2 T of full fat sour cream	spinach salad
1 cup of creamed spinach	1 T of vinaigrette
Calories: 915 Fat: 54	Calories: 471 Fat: 14

The payoff:

◄ Substituting the beef with 3 oz of pork saves 233 calories and reduces fat by 13 grams.

◄ Substituting the baked potato with a sweet potato is a huge antioxidant boost.

◄ Substituting the full-fat butter and sour cream with the low-fat versions saves 110 calories and reduces fat by 13 grams.

◄ Substituting the creamed spinach with a small spinach salad boosts the veggie servings, saves 101 calories, and reduces fat by 14 grams.

◄ This makeover saves 444 calories, increases the veggie servings to 4, reduces fat by 42 grams, and adds a huge antioxidant boost!

Okay, Let's Review:

◄ Most meals can be made healthier and with fewer calories by making better food choices and adhering to the standard serving size within the various food groups.

◄ By making healthier food choices, you can trade empty calories for calories packed with fiber, vitamins, minerals, antioxidants, and phytochemicals.

◄ Making a few simple changes in your diet can provide a huge payoff in making you healthier and maintaining your weight for life.

Note to self:
I'm going to give my tired old fattening meals a nutrition makeover so I can be healthier and slimmer.

In Section 2, The Simple Nutrition Meal Plan, you'll see how easy it is to follow a nutritious eating plan, without giving up taste!

The Simple Nutrition ▶ Meal Plan

Multi-Task Meals and More

So far, we've given you the 411 on the stuff you need to make better lifestyle choices—the most important rules of nutrition coupled with sound weight loss strategies. Now to stay true to our name, "Simple Nutrition," we want to make things super easy for you by providing our top-notch meals on a silver platter! We call them Multi-task Meals. Our meals were designed by professionals and they include the healthiest foods, along with portion and calorie control, in an easy-to-follow format. Our goal is to help make healthy eating a part of your daily lifestyle!

Why The Multi-Task Meal Concept?

That's easy. As women, we have the innate ability to "multi-task" in most areas of our daily lives. For many, this special ability starts at a young age. For instance, in school we begin to hone our multi-tasking skills by learning to study for exams in the library while keenly scoping out a date for Saturday night. As we blossom into career women, we begin to juggle more tasks simultaneously—we can work on a presentation to the board of directors and talk to a friend in need, both while making happy hour plans, via e-mail, with our man du jour. All this without missing a beat! As wives and mothers, we take these multi-tasking skills to a completely new level. Not only do many of us bring home the bacon, and fry it up in a pan, but we proceed to serve it up, clean it up, do a couple loads of laundry, pick up, and get the kids bathed and to bed. Then comes the relaxing part—preparing for the next day so we can do it all over again! And of course, as the song goes, we are capable of doing all of this because we're women ("I'm a woman, w-o-m-a-n"). Yeah, whatever.

With **The Simple Nutrition Meal Plan**, we'll show you how to put these God-given "multi-tasking" skills to even better use so you can enjoy **A Better Body, Better Health, and a Better Life!** Intrigued? Read on.

What Exactly Is A Multi-Task Meal?

The official definition of a **Multi-task Meal** is a meal that provides as many health benefits as possible—at one time. More specifically, our **Multi-task Meals** provide most or all of these things:

- ◄ **Great taste while packing a nutritional punch**
- ◄ **Disease-fighting foods**
- ◄ **Anti-aging properties**
- ◄ **Proper portions and calorie control**
- ◄ **A combo of whole grains, quality protein, and good fat**
- ◄ **Mainly whole foods** (with minimal processed foods)
- ◄ **Multiple servings of fruits or veggies**
- ◄ **High-fiber foods**
- ◄ **No trans fats**
- ◄ **Easy preparation and fast cleanup**

You're probably asking yourself how in the world these meals can pack this kind of nutritional punch and still be easy to prepare. It sounds daunting, but when you see how easy it is to incorporate the **Multi-task Meal** concept into your new eating plan, you'll be hooked for life! What follows are the two simple steps we took to create this unique meal plan.

First, we created our list of the top 21 nutritional powerhouse foods that make up the superstars from each of the five food groups. What's key about this list is that these foods are not obscure, hard-to-find items. You'll find them in almost every grocery store, anywhere. Take a look at these powerhouse foods on the next page.

▶

Top 21 Powerhouse Foods

We chose these 21 foods listed in the chart below because they are each packed with vitamins, minerals, antioxidants, and phytochemicals—all of which have the power to help keep you healthy, prevent chronic diseases, and keep you slim!

Whole Grains
High-fiber cereal (10 grams or more)
Whole-wheat pasta
Whole-wheat bread

Fruits
Berries (especially blueberries)
Kiwi
Avocado
Cantaloupe

Veggies
Crucifers (broccoli, cauliflower, kale)
Spinach
Lycopenes (tomatoes, tomato sauce, salsa)
Carrots

Meat/Alternatives
Salmon
Tuna
Beans (black beans, chickpeas, kidney)
Peanut butter (all natural)
Walnuts

Dairy
Skim milk
Low-fat yogurt
Calcium fortified orange juice

Other
Green tea
Dark chocolate

The goal is to include as many of these foods into your daily diet as possible, and that's where the second step of our unique plan comes into play. Next, we took a handful of meal staples, like salads, sandwiches, pasta dishes, egg dishes, stir-frys, etc., and began the multitasking process by adding as many powerhouse foods to each meal as possible.

On the next page, we'll show you a sample menu and how we easily included 15 out of the 21 powerhouse foods in these basic meals!

Sample Menu of Powerhouse Foods

Breakfast: We took a basic cereal meal and turned it into a Multi-task Meal by choosing a high-fiber cereal (we like Fiber One because it packs a whopping 14 grams of fiber in 1 serving). Next, we added 1 serving of skim milk, and then topped it off with 1 serving each of blueberries and a banana. This meal provides 50% of the daily fiber requirement and satisfies the **following servings: 1 grain, 2 fruits, and 1 dairy. Prep time: less than one minute!**

Lunch: We took a basic salad meal and turned it into a Multi-task Meal by including a serving each of the following: baby spinach leaves, shredded carrots, diced tomatoes, black beans, chopped walnuts, and shredded low fat mozzarella. We topped it off with 2 tablespoons of vinaigrette, served it with a whole-wheat roll and a glass of calcium fortified orange juice. This meal is jam-packed with fiber, antioxidants, and phytochemicals, and satisfies the **following servings: 1 grain, 3 veggies, 2 meat alternatives, and 1 dairy. Prep time: less than two minutes!**

Snack: We took a basic snack of an apple and turned it into a Multi-task Meal by adding 1 serving of low fat yogurt and 1 serving of whole-wheat crackers. This snack satisfies the **following servings: 1 grain, 1 fruit, and 1 dairy. Prep time: less than 1 minute.**

Dinner: We took a basic pasta dish and turned it into a Multi-task Meal by including a serving of lean ground beef and sautéing it with 1 serving each of shitake mushrooms and spinach. We combined a serving of tomato and basil sauce (from the jar) with the meat mixture, added it to 1 cup of cooked whole-wheat spaghetti noodles, served it with 1 piece of whole-wheat garlic bread, and a cup of green tea. This meal satisfies the **following servings: 3 grains, 3 veggies, and 1 meat. Prep time: less than 3 minutes; Cook time: about 15 minutes.**

Okay, combine these four meals over the course of a day, and here's what you get:

Approximate calories:	**1,600**
Whole-grain servings:	6
Fruit servings:	3
Veggie servings:	6
Meat/alternatives servings:	3
Dairy servings:	3
Total prep time:	Less than 10 minutes
Health benefits:	Priceless!

▶

Eating Well Is the Best Revenge!

Now you see how easy it can be to pack these powerhouse foods into your daily meals with minimal prep time! The trick is having them on hand so that you can create your own Multi-task Meals by adding as many of these foods as possible (with an emphasis on the fruits and veggies) to your basic meals. The result will be top-notch, nutritious meals that are easy to prepare, with health benefits that are priceless!

Now that you understand the Multi-task Meal concept, we're ready to provide everything you need to get started! On the pages that follow, you'll find our Simple Nutrition Meal Plan that includes a variety of meal choices, along with The Ultimate Shopping List. Getting healthy and slim has never been so easy—and yummy!

The Simple Nutrition Meal Plan

The Simple Nutrition Meal Plan provides everything you need to customize an eating plan based on your personal goals. Whether you're just in it for some new, healthy meal suggestions, or you're in need of a complete nutrition makeover, we can help! Here's what you'll find with our meal plan:

◄ A variety of Multi-task Meal options for breakfast, lunch, dinner, snacks, and dessert (yes, even dessert).

◄ Meals that take little time to prepare, because we offer simple variety and include many food items that can be purchased "ready to eat"—like veggies that are precut, shredded, and washed, and dairy items that come packaged in single servings for easy portion control.

◄ A list of all the ingredients for each meal along with their portion sizes and calorie counts. This allows for easy mixing and matching of meals; you'll quickly learn the standard portion sizes and calorie counts for these powerhouse foods!

◄ A listing of the food groups that are represented for each meal to help you track your daily nutrition goals.

- ◄ Recipes and instructions for preparing meals , where needed.

- ◄ A shopping list that includes every food item from each meal, along with our favorite brand suggestions, to make shopping a breeze!

Our Easy-To-Follow Plan

In addition to being super healthy, our meal plan is exceptionally easy to follow too. Here's how it works: Each day, you can choose one meal from each of the columns, breakfast (each meal is about 300 calories), lunch (about 400 calories), dinner (about 500 calories), snacks (about 200 calories), and dessert (about 100 calories). Altogether, that totals about 1,600 calories per day.

If your daily calorie budget* is above or below 1,600 calories per day, simply add or subtract meals (or ingredients from the meals you choose) in order to customize the plan to meet your personal goals.

In the beginning, we suggest not varying your weekly meals too much. Instead, be a repeat offender of healthy meals! For instance, you might want to choose two meal options each for breakfast, lunch, dinner, and snacks and repeat these most days over the course of the week. The repetition of the meals makes it easier to shop, stick to your plan, and track calories; it also helps to create healthy lifestyle habits. Since variety is important, you can incorporate different meals week-to-week—but, again, repeat these new meals over the course of that specific week.

You'll see that it won't take long to master our Multi-task Meal concept. Once you do, you may want to venture out and experiment with different recipes and even more variety, because you'll have all the tools and information right at your fingertips to create your own well-balanced meals! Turn the page to take a look at our tasty meals!

* In Section 3, we'll walk you through a series of worksheets that will help you create your personal makeover plan, which includes determining your personal calorie budget.

▶

The Simple Nutrition Meals

Note: If you are preparing meals for others in addition to yourself, multiply the quantities shown by the number of people served.

To follow the plan, simply choose from the list of meals below for breakfast, lunch, dinner, snacks, and dessert. Since we list all of the ingredients for each meal along with the portion sizes and approximate calorie counts, you can easily mix and match these meals to fit your personal preferences.

Be sure to check out our no-fail planning, organizing, and tracking system in Section 4, **The Simple Nutrition Organizer.** We'll show you how to begin incorporating these tasty meals into your daily life by using the weekly meal planning and grocery list sheets. Plus, you can track your progress on the daily journal sheets. With this "day timer" format, being healthy and slim has never been so easy!

Multi-Task Meals for Breakfast (about 300 calories)

Cereal*

¾ cup of high-fiber cereal	90
1 cup of skim milk	90
1 small banana	105
½ cup of blueberries	40
Total Calories:	**325**

__1.5__ Grains __2__ Fruits/Veggies __0__ Meat/Alternatives __1__ Dairy

*We recommend the high-fiber cereal meal most mornings, because it's a great way to get **more than 50%** of your daily fiber in one meal. Since variety is the spice of life, we included other nutritious breakfast options for you to choose from when you need a change.

Yogurt Mixture

1 cup of low-fat plain yogurt	130
1 diced kiwi	45
½ cup of strawberries	40
2 T of walnuts	100
Total Calories:	**315**

__0__ Grains __2__ Fruits/Veggies __½__ Meat/Alternatives __1__ Dairy

Bagel

½ whole-wheat bagel (small)	80
1 T of low-fat cream cheese	35
1 cup of cantaloupe	60
6 oz glass of OJ (calcium fortified)*	90
Total Calories:	**265**

__1__ Grains __2__ Fruits/Veggies __0__ Meat/Alternatives __1__ Dairy

*Note: Calcium fortified orange juice counts as a fruit serving and a dairy serving—it's a double whammy!

Omelet*

3 egg whites	70
1 cup of sautéed veggies	60
2 T of low-fat cheddar cheese	40
4 T of salsa	20
1 slice of whole-wheat toast	80
Total Calories:	**270**

__1__ Grains __3__ Fruits/Veggies __2__ Meat/Alternatives __½__ Dairy

*You can include onions, fresh spinach, tomatoes, mushrooms, and peppers and top with cheddar cheese and salsa.

Oatmeal

½ cup of slow-cooking oatmeal	80
1 cup of skim milk (mix with oatmeal)	90
½ cup of blueberries	40
6 oz glass of OJ (calcium fortified)	90
1 tsp of butter*	—-
1 T of brown sugar*	—-
Total Calories:	**300**

__1__ Grains   __2__ Fruits/Veggies   __0__ Meat/Alternatives   __1__ Dairy

*Optional, add an extra 65 calories.

Smoothie*

1 small banana	105
½ cup of frozen strawberries	40
1 tsp of peanut butter	50
½ cup of low-fat yogurt	75
6 oz glass of OJ (calcium fortified)	90
Total Calories:	**360**

__0__ Grains   __3__ Fruits/Veggies   __0__ Meat/Alternatives   __1½__ Dairy

* Blend all ingredients until liquefied.

Tip: We recommend that you choose water as your beverage of choice with most meals. It will help satisfy your daily water goal and is calorie-free!

Tuna Pita*

1 whole-wheat pita (6 ½")	130
3 oz of tuna packed in water	90
1 chopped apple	60
1 chopped celery piece	5
1 T of Dijon mustard	5
4 T of low-fat shredded mozzarella	80
½ cup of baby carrots	30
Total Calories:	**400**

 2 Grains   **2** Fruits/Veggies   **1** Meat/Alternatives **1** Dairy

* Drain tuna; mix with Dijon mustard, chopped apple, and chopped celery. Season to taste with black pepper. Fill pita with tuna mixture and top with mozzarella cheese. Serve with baby carrots.

Egg Salad Sandwich*

2 slices of whole-wheat bread	160
3 egg whites, 1 yolk	110
1 T of Dijon mustard	5
½ cup of chopped red peppers	25
1 cup of baby spinach leaves	10
1 tsp of capers	35
½ cup of baby carrots	30
7 organic tortilla chips	75
Total Calories:	**450**

 3 Grains   **3** Fruits/Veggies   **1** Meat/Alternatives **0** Dairy

*Boil eggs and let cool for 15 minutes; discard two yolks. Mix eggs with Dijon mustard, chopped red peppers, and capers. Make sandwich with egg mixture and spinach leaves. Serve with the chips and baby carrots.

▶

Soup and Sandwich

1 cup of lentil soup	120
½ whole-wheat pita (6½")	65
1 ½ oz of turkey	50
½ cup of baby spinach leaves	5
1 tomato slice	15
2 T of shredded low fat mozzarella	40
1 T vinaigrette	35
1 apple	60
Total Calories:	**390**

3 Grains **1½** Fruits/Veggies **1½** Meat/Alternatives **½** Dairy

Spinach Salad

2 cups of baby spinach	20
½ cup of shredded carrots	30
1 diced tomato	25
½ cup of black beans	100
1 T of chopped walnuts	50
2 T of shredded low fat mozzarella	40
2 T of balsamic vinaigrette	70
1 small whole-wheat roll	80
Total Calories:	**415**

1 Grains **4** Fruits/Veggies **1** Meat/Alternatives **½** Dairy

Tip: When choosing fruits and veggies, you have some options. There's fresh, frozen, canned, or dried. Fresh is usually best, but frozen is a close second because they are usually just as nutritious, they last longer, and they're less expensive! Canned and dried are good options too, but watch out for the high sodium content!

Stuffed Sweet Potato & Salad

1 small sweet potato	120
½ cup of low fat cottage cheese	80
2 T of raw sunflower seeds	100
1 small spinach salad (mixed veggies)**	60
1 T of vinaigrette	35
Total Calories:	**395**

0 Grains   **4** Fruits/Veggies   **1** Meat/Alternatives   **0** Dairy

Fruit Salad

1 cup of low-fat cottage cheese	135
½ cup of blueberries	40
1 kiwi	45
2 T of walnuts	100
5 whole-wheat crackers	80
Total Calories:	**400**

1 Grains   **2** Fruits/Veggies   **1½** Meat/Alternatives   **½** Dairy

Veggie Tacos*

½ cup of black beans (rinsed and heated)	100
½ cup of cooked brown rice	80
2 T of low fat sour cream	45
4 T of salsa	20
2 corn tortillas (warmed)	100
¼ cup of diced avocado	80
½ cup of grape tomatoes	20
7 organic tortilla chips	75
Total Calories:	**520**

3 Grains   **2.5** Fruits/Veggies   **1** Meat/Alternatives   **0** Dairy

*Mix cooked beans and rice together. Spoon into warmed corn tortillas and top with avocado, tomatoes, sour cream, and salsa. Warm tortillas between two small plates in the microwave for about 10-15 seconds.

Spaghetti with Meat Sauce

1 cup of cooked whole-wheat spaghetti	160
½ cup of lean ground beef	165
½ cup of tomato sauce (jar)	80
2 tsp of grated Parmesan cheese	25
1 small spinach salad (mixed veggies)**	60
1 T of vinaigrette	35
Total Calories:	**525**

__2__ Grains __4__ Fruits/Veggies __1__ Meat/Alternatives __0__ Dairy

Shrimp Stir-Fry*

6 medium shrimp	90
1 tsp of olive oil	60
2 cups of frozen veggies	100
2 T of peanut sauce	80
½ cup of brown rice	80
1 T of raw almonds	50
Total Calories:	**460**

__1__ Grains __2__ Fruits/Veggies __1__ Meat/Alternatives __0__ Dairy

*Sauté shrimp in a lightly oiled, nonstick skillet over medium heat for 6 to 8 minutes or until cooked through. Add frozen veggies (broccoli, carrots, red peppers, and snow peas). Cook until veggies are tender (don't overcook). Toss with peanut sauce. Serve over rice and top with almonds.

**A small spinach salad is 1 cup of baby spinach, with ½ cup of shredded carrots, and 1-diced Roma tomato.

Baked Salmon*

3 oz of baked salmon	155
1 tsp of olive oil	60
1 T of paprika	—-
1 cup of steamed broccoli	50
1 tsp of butter	45
1 spinach salad (mixed veggies)	60
1 T of walnuts (add to salad)	50
1 T vinaigrette	40
½ cup of brown rice	80
Total Calories:	**540**

__1__ Grains __5__ Fruits/Veggies __1__ Meat/Alternatives __0__ Dairy

*Brush salmon with 1 tsp of olive oil and season with paprika on both sides. Bake for 15 minutes at 350° or until cooked through. Serve with broccoli, small spinach salad, and rice.

Pork Tenderloin*

3 oz of baked pork tenderloin	165
1 small sweet potato	120
2 T of low-fat sour cream	45
1 cup of sautéed spinach	50
1 tsp of olive oil	60
1 small whole-wheat roll	80
Total Calories:	**520**

__1__ Grains __3__ Fruits/Veggies __1__ Meat/Alternatives __0__ Dairy

* Use pre-marinated pork tenderloin and bake according to directions along with the sweet potato. Heat nonstick skillet with the olive oil and sauté spinach until tender.

Pasta Salad (served cold)*

1 cup of cooked whole-wheat pasta (bow tie)	160
½ cup of kidney beans	120
½ cup of grape tomatoes	30
½ cup of red grapes	20
½ cup of broccoli	25
1 T of walnuts	50
1 T of feta cheese	40
2 T of vinaigrette	70
Total Calories:	**515**

2 Grains **3** Fruits/Veggies **1** Meat/Alternatives **0** Dairy

*Mix beans, tomatoes, grapes, and broccoli with pasta. Stir in vinaigrette and mix well, then chill for one hour. Top with feta cheese and walnuts.

Multi-Task Snacks (about 200 calories each)

Yogurt

½ cup of low-fat yogurt	110
1 T of walnuts	50
1 cup of red grapes	60
Total Calories:	**220**

0 Grains **2** Fruits/Veggies **0** Meat/Alternatives **½** Dairy

Cottage Cheese

½ cup of low-fat cottage cheese	80
1 T of almonds	50
1 kiwi	60
Total Calories:	**190**

0 Grains **1** Fruits/Veggies **½** Meat/Alternatives **0** Dairy

Cheese and Crackers

1 single serving of string cheese	80
1 cup of baby carrots	60
5 medium whole-wheat crackers	80
Total Calories:	**220**

1 Grains **2** Fruits/Veggies **0** Meat/Alternatives **1** Dairy

Apple and Peanut Butter

1 apple	80
1 T of all natural peanut butter	100
Total Calories:	**180**

0 Grains **1** Fruits/Veggies **½** Meat/Alternatives **0** Dairy

Hard-Boiled Eggs and Carrots

1 hard-boiled egg	75
1 cup of baby carrots	60
4 T of salsa	20
Total Calories:	**155**

0 Grains **3** Fruits/Veggies **1** Meat/Alternatives **0** Dairy

Hummus and Pita

½ cup of hummus	120
½ whole-wheat pita (6 ½")	65
1 cup of baby carrots	60
Total Calories:	**245**

½ Grains **2** Fruits/Veggies **½** Meat/Alternatives **0** Dairy

Chips and Salsa

7 organic tortilla chips	75
4 T of salsa	20
½ diced avocado	80
Total Calories:	**175**

1 Grains **2** Fruits/Veggie **0** Meat/Alternatives **0** Dairy

Desserts (about 100 calories)

2 small pieces of dark chocolate	90
½ cup of pudding	110
1 small fudgsicle	90
2 fig cookies	90
7 animal crackers	90
1 packet of instant hot chocolate	50
½ cup of low-fat frozen yogurt	125
½ cup of low-fat ice cream	100
2 graham cracker squares with 1 tsp of peanut butter	100

Extras (about 50 calories)

1 tsp of butter	35
1 T of brown sugar	25
1 T of low-fat sour cream	25
1 T low-fat cream cheese	35
2 T of salsa	10
1 T of balsamic vinaigrette	35
1 spinach salad*	60
½ oz of organic tortilla chips**	75

*1 cup of spinach, ½ cup of shredded carrots, and 1 diced Roma tomato.
** ½ oz of tortilla chips is about 7 medium-sized chips.

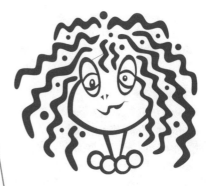

Note from Mom:
If you can't get
your man on The
Simple Nutrition
Meal Plan, then
make sure he at
least has a big life
insurance policy.
*There's always a
silver lining!*

Let's go shopping! On the next page, you'll find The Ultimate Shopping List that includes every food item listed in our meal plan to make shopping a breeze.

Below we've compiled a master list of all the food items for each of the suggested meals in our plan. Where appropriate, we've inserted our **favorite brand** to help make shopping a breeze (our favorites are in purple). Be sure to check out our comprehensive list by food group of "Best Brands" in Section 4, for other brand options.

Whole Grains

General Mills Fiber One cereal
Toufayan Whole Wheat Pita
Hodgson Mill Whole Wheat Spaghetti
Kashi TLC Whole Grain Crackers
Cobblestone Mill 100% Whole Wheat Bread

Earth Grains Cinnamon Raisin Bagels
Success 10 Minute Instant Brown Rice
Corn tortillas

Produce

Cantaloupe
Kiwi
Bananas
Earthbound Farm Organic Baby Spinach
Avocados
Apples
Seedless red grapes
Red bell peppers

Onions
Shitake mushrooms
Shredded carrots
Sweet potatoes
Roma tomatoes
Grape tomatoes
Zucchini
Baby carrots

Frozen

Cascadian Farm Blueberries
Cascadian Farm Strawberries
Cascadian Farm Broccoli Cuts
Frozen stir-fry veggie medley

Meat/Fish/Poultry

Salmon fillets
Hormel Pork Tenderloin
Lean ground beef
Skinless chicken breasts
Contessa Frozen Cooked Shrimp
Contessa Stir-Fry Shrimp Dinner
Athenos Hummus
Boar's Head Turkey Breast

Canned/Packaged Goods

Canned water-packed tuna

Smucker's Natural Peanut Butter

Jam

Raw almonds

Raw walnuts

Raw cashews

Raw sunflower seeds

Progresso Lentil Soup

Dijon mustard

Wish-Bone Balsamic Vinaigrette

Bertolli Tomato & Basil Sauce

Tostitos All Natural Salsa

Peanut sauce

Capers

Black beans, kidney beans, and chickpeas

Olive oil

Brown sugar

Paprika

Garden of Eatin' Blue Chips (organic tortilla chips)

Barbara's Bakery Organic Go Go Graham Crackers

Fig Newman's (Newman's Own)

Newman's Own Alphabet Cookies

Pudding

Fudgsicles

Dove Dark Promises

Instant hot chocolate (no sugar added)

Low-fat ice cream

Dairy

Skim milk

Low-fat soymilk

Butter

Stoneyfield Farm Lowfat Plain Yogurt

Low-fat cottage cheese

String cheese

Jarlsberg Lite Swiss Cheese

Shredded part-skim mozzarella cheese

Shredded low-fat cheddar cheese

Low-fat feta cheese

Parmesan cheese

Eggs

Low-fat sour cream

Low-fat cream cheese

Low-fat frozen yogurt

Low-fat ice cream

Orange juice (calcium fortified)

Miscellaneous

Lipton Flavored Green Tea

Bottled water

Tupperware

Plastic bags (small and big for storing)

In Section 3, Designing Your Personal Makeover Plan, you'll create an action plan for incorporating these healthy meals into your daily lifestyle!

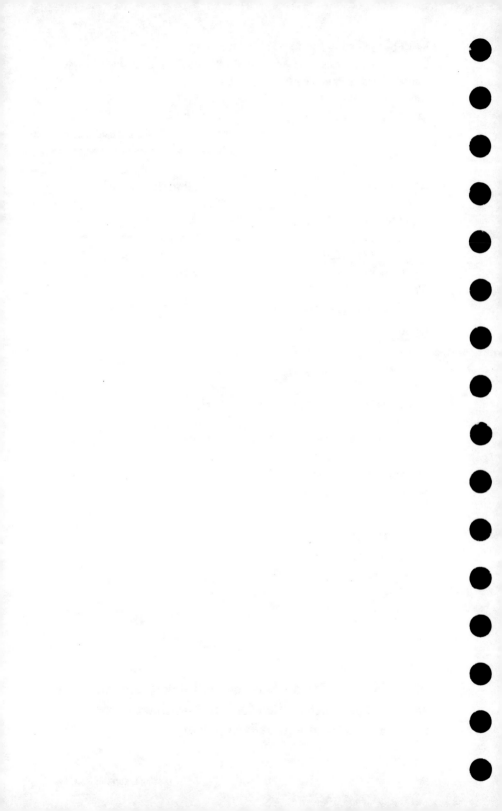

The Simple Nutrition ▶ Makeover Plan

Section 3

Chapter 8

Designing Your
Personal Makeover Plan

Things we'll cover in this chapter:	▶ Why planning is key for weight loss
	▶ Our two phase program
	▶ Personal Calorie Budget Worksheet
	▶ Healthy Habits Worksheet
	▶ Personal Makeover Plan Worksheet

Okay, let's recap. We've laughed, we've cried. We know a healthy diet from an unhealthy one, and that eating well is the best revenge! We know the good fats from the bad and that we should avoid the ugly fats at all costs! We know the benefits of downsizing our meals rather than supersizing them, and we can detect an unhealthy food label from a mile away. Now what?

Well, it's time to get down to the nitty gritty of creating an eating and lifestyle plan fit for the real world—**yours.** In this planning section, we'll walk you through several worksheets that are designed to provide very specific information about you that will be used to create your personal makeover plan for success! For instance, once you've completed the worksheets, you'll have the following:

◄ **An action plan that outlines your personal health and weight loss goals.**

◄ **The steps you'll take to reach these goals.**

◄ **A timeline for accomplishing your goals.**

Before you begin filling out your planning worksheets, we think it's important for you to understand why having a plan is a key component to achieving permanent weight loss. Read on.

Planning Is Key To Permanent Weight Loss

"Plan your work, work your plan." "If you fail to plan, your plan will fail." We've heard these age-old adages repeatedly over the course of our lives. Why? Because they're true. If you have a goal, the best way to achieve it is to have an action plan. Think about it. We plan our shopping excursions to ensure that we'll hit all the hot spots and catch all the sales to acquire the latest and greatest fashions at the best prices. We plan social engagements weeks in advance; most of us know what we're doing every Saturday night for the next month. We plan vacations down to the last detail. We know the restaurants we'll visit, the outfits we'll wear, and what sites we'll see.

So shouldn't we also create a plan for our nutrition and weight loss goals? Of course we should. At the end of the day, having your health and being within a healthy weight range is everything. Not to mention that being at your "fighting weight" makes shopping, socializing, vacationing, and life in general a whole lot more enjoyable!

Our Two Phase Program

Okay, ladies, time to focus. Here's where we'll briefly walk you through the two phases necessary for designing and implementing your new makeover plan. Once you've reviewed the information, all you'll need is the motivation and desire to make a few lifestyle changes and a pencil to complete the planning worksheets! That's it.

The Planning Phase

1. Read Section 1, Simple Nutrition 101 (if you haven't already done so). This is imperative because, although you do not have to memorize all of the nutritional and weight loss information, you do need to have a general understanding of how it works, why it works, and the overall benefits to your health.

2. Complete the Unhealthy Habits Survey. This survey will help you analyze your current situation, determine the areas where you need to make changes, provide healthy replacements for your unhealthy habits, and will help you to create a plan you can live with.

3. Create a Calorie Budget. This planning sheet will walk you through the simple steps you'll need to determine a safe yet effective calorie budget that will be instrumental in helping you to maintain or lose weight.

4. Complete Your Personal Makeover Plan Worksheet. This is where you will actually document your goals in writing, decide how to reach them, and then set a realistic target date for achieving them.

This ends the planning phase. The next phase is where you'll actually implement your action plan with our easy-to-use activity sheets found in Section 4 (the day-timer portion).

The Implementation Phase

5. Review the Multi-Task Meal Selections in Section 2 (if you haven't already done so). This is the fun part where you decide which foods and meals you will incorporate into your new eating plan!

6. Fill Out Your Weekly Meal and Exercise Worksheet. This is where you plan your meals and exercise for each day within a given week. Having a plan to refer back to will help keep you on track. We provide 8 weeks worth of these sheets because we think that will give you enough time to develop a plan that you can follow for life.

7. Create Your Weekly Grocery List Sheet. You will complete this sheet based upon the meals you choose each week. Making a grocery list will ensure that you stock your fridge with healthy food choices!

8. Document Your Progress on Your Daily Makeover Journal Sheets. This is where you write down EVERYTHING you actually eat each day, along with your exercise, to help keep you honest. At the end of each week, you can chart your overall progress and determine where you need to tweak your plan and set new goals for the next week.

Are you ready to create your personal makeover plan? Then fasten your seatbelts; the real fun is about to begin! Your next step will be to take the Unhealthy Habits Survey. The results of this survey will be instrumental in helping you to meet your nutrition and weight loss goals.

Here's where you'll come to terms with your current lifestyle habits. This includes looking at your eating, exercise, and overall nutrition habits. This worksheet is designed to do the following:

Analyze your current lifestyle—sometimes seeing your bad habits on paper can really hit home.

Pinpoint the areas where you need to make changes—knowing what needs to be changed is half the battle.

Provide healthier choices for your unhealthy habits—the other half of the battle is knowing what changes to make.

Help you to create a plan you can live with—without a personalized plan, you probably won't stick with it.

In order to complete this worksheet, follow these three easy steps:

Step 1:
Complete the Unhealthy Habits Survey.

Step 2:
Add up your points to determine your lifestyle score.

Step 3:
Complete the Healthy Habits section.

Step 1: Unhealthy Habits Survey

On the next page, you'll find five categories of unhealthy habits. For each statement that describes you, put the number of points indicated for each category in the left-hand column; if it doesn't apply to you, leave the space blank. It's important to really be honest here. No one is going to judge you; this can only help you to create better habits going forward. If your pencil is sharpened, then turn the page to begin!

General Habits (Add 2 points for each statement that describes you.)

_____I do not consistently take a multivitamin.

_____I do not receive annual routine medical exams appropriate for my age.

_____I do not understand the role nutrition plays in preventing diseases.

_____I do not have a nutritional and weight management plan.

_____I very rarely, if ever, plan my meals daily or weekly.

_____I do not stock my fridge with healthy foods; I usually buy junk food.

_____I have a "wing-it" mentality when ordering food in restaurants.

_____I have no idea how many calories I consume on average each day.

Meal/Snack Habits (Add 2 points for each statement that describes you.)

_____My diet consists mostly of processed foods, especially fast food.

_____I often skip breakfast.

_____I often skip meals and then binge because I'm starving.

_____I rarely incorporate healthy snacks into my day.

Portion Habits (Add 2 points for each statement that best describes you.)

_____I tend to supersize when I eat fast food.

_____I usually eat everything on my plate when dining out.

_____I do not know how to eyeball a standard serving for any of the food groups.

Nutritional Habits (Add 3 points for each statement that best describes you.)

_____I do not eat 5 to 10 fruits and veggies each day.

_____I have no idea if I eat the recommended servings from the food groups.

_____I have no idea what the ingredients are in the foods that I consume.

_____I am not sure if I get enough good fat in my diet.

_____I do not know how much trans fat I consume.

_____I do not eat low-fat versions of meat and dairy products.

_____I have no idea if I eat enough fiber.

_____I try to avoid all carbs because I think they make me fat.

_____I drink mostly sodas, coffee, fruit drinks, or sweet tea throughout the day.

_____I do not drink 8 glasses of water each day.

Exercise Habits (Add 5 points for each statement that best describes you.)

_____I do not consistently exercise.

_____I do not have time to exercise.

_____I exercise less than three times per week for less than 30 minutes each time.

Add up your points from the Unhealthy Habits Survey to determine your lifestyle score. Then see how you rate below.

My Lifestyle Score_____.

0-4 Points (Well above average)

Congratulations! Overall, you have very good lifestyle habits! You obviously take good care of yourself through healthy eating habits and consistent exercise, which will pay dividends to you over the long run in terms of your health and weight management.

5-10 Points (Average)

Don't Panic! Your lifestyle habits are about average, but there is always room for improvement. After all, you do not want to be just average, do you? We recommend that you focus on acquiring a few new healthy habits. If you make just a few small changes, you will see a significant difference in your overall health and weight loss goals. Don't reinvent the wheel; refer to our list of healthy habits located on the next page!

11-20 Points (Below average)

Gulp! Your lifestyle habits are below average and it's time to think about a lifestyle makeover! Making positive changes does not mean an all-or-nothing approach. It's more about moderation. Healthy lifestyle habits are really pretty simple; it's just a matter of knowing what they are and how to easily incorporate them into your everyday life. The lifestyle suggestions listed in this section will help you through the transition.

21-28 Points (Well below average)

Can we talk? There's no way to sugarcoat it—you are in a full blown unhealthy lifestyle habit rut! Even if you are not suffering any adverse effects now, you are on the fast track to disease and being overweight. We recommend that you focus on **the payoffs** for incorporating healthy habits into your daily life to help get you motivated to make some important and very necessary changes in your lifestyle. The healthy lifestyle suggestions listed in this section will help you through the transition. Time is of the essence; start today!

The worst part is over. You know where you stand. Now it's time to trade in those bad habits for more healthy habits that will help you achieve the three B's— A Better Body, Better Health, and a Better Life! Review each statement below and check off the healthy habit that is associated with the unhealthy habit you checked off in Step 1. These new, healthy habits will be the basis of your Personal Makeover Plan Worksheet.

General Habits

_____ I will begin consistently taking a multivitamin with folate every day.

_____ I will make appointments to receive annual routine medical exams.

_____ I will make an effort to understand how nutrition helps prevent diseases.

_____ I will create a nutritional/weight loss action plan that I can follow for life.

_____ I will begin planning my meals each week.

_____ I will stock my fridge with healthy foods and avoid buying junk food.

_____ I will make healthier choices when ordering out.

_____ I will begin to record my daily meals and exercise in a journal.

Meal/Snack Habits

_____ I will limit my fast-food consumption.

_____ I will incorporate whole foods into my diet by cutting back on processed foods.

_____ I will eat a healthy breakfast every day.

_____ I will eat 5 to 6 mini-meals each day to avoid binge eating.

_____ I will eat healthy snacks every day by keeping them handy.

Portion Habits

_____ I will avoid supersizing when I eat out and adhere to standard serving sizes.

_____ I will follow the Dining-Out Tips on page 212 in order to control my portions.

_____ I will learn how to eyeball standard serving sizes for the major food groups.

Nutritional Habits

_____ I will incorporate more fruits and veggies at each meal.

_____ I will eat a variety of foods from the major food groups each day.

_____ I will look at food labels in order to avoid eating unhealthy ingredients.

_____ I will include "good fats" at each meal to help me feel fuller.

_____ I will avoid processed foods that contain trans fats whenever possible.

_____ I will choose low-fat versions of meat and dairy products.

_____ I will reach my fiber goal each day by increasing fruits/veggies, whole grains, and incorporating a high-fiber cereal into my diet.

_____ I will not eliminate whole grain carbs, because they are essential for good health.

_____ I will limit my intake of soda, coffee, fruit drinks, and sweet tea.

_____ I will make it a priority to drink at least 8 glasses of water every day.

Exercise Habits

_____ I will consistently exercise for at least 30 minutes most days.

_____ I will make time to exercise most days.

_____ I will increase my exercise to at least five times per week, for a minimum of 30 minutes each time.

You now have your "hit list" of healthy habits identified; these will be used to help create your Personal Makeover Plan. Don't you feel better already?

It is a simple and undeniable fact that calories do count when it comes to weight loss! Even though we constantly hear about fad diets that claim calories **don't** matter, upon further inspection, you'll find the real reason these types of diets work is because dieters lowered their calorie intake! In other words, they created a calorie deficit that led to weight loss.

In this worksheet, we're going to show you how to create a realistic calorie deficit that will help you to lose weight the good old fashion way—by eating less and exercising more. The process involves three easy steps. They include:

Step 1:
Create a personal daily calorie budget.

Step 2:
Create a personal weekly calorie expenditure budget.

Step 3:
Determine the number of servings you'll need from the major food groups.

Before we begin, we need to address a very touchy subject—MATH. Read on at your own risk.

"You Do the Math"!

No, this time we really mean it. You'll actually need to do the math in this section to figure out the calorie deficit needed to reach your weight loss goals. We don't mean calculus, trigonometry, or anything scary like that, just plain old adding, subtracting and multiplying. For those of you that have a math phobia we thought it best to get this touchy subject out of the way from the get-go. But here's some good news. We absolutely insist that you use a calculator. You may now breathe a sigh of relief.

Simple Formula For Losing Weight

Before you begin filling out your Calorie Budget/Expenditure Worksheets, we think it's important for you to really understand how this whole calorie deficit thing works, because when it comes to permanent weight loss—calories count, bottom line.

First, most health professionals recommend slow weight loss as the safest and most effective approach. This equates to about 1 to 2 pounds per week. This type of gradual weight loss promotes long—term loss of body fat—not just water weight that can be easily gained back.   Okay, but how do we actually lose 1 to 2 pounds per week? It's simple:

Burn More Calories Than You Take In!

Here's the skinny: In order to lose just 1 pound, a person must burn 3,500 calories __more__ than are consumed over the course of one week (which is about 500 calories per day). There are two ways to create this type of calorie deficit: eat fewer calories or burn more calories. We think the best strategy for achieving permanent weight loss is to do both.

Here's an example of how that can be done:

Say you need to eat 2,000 calories a day to maintain your weight, but want to lose. You'll need to cut 500 calories from your daily calorie budget to lose 1 pound a week. To do this, you could reduce your calories by just 300 per day (that's like a medium-sized cookie and a 12 oz soda) and increase your exercise to burn off an additional 200 calories. If you did this each day for seven days, you would lose 1 pound by week's end. If you wanted to lose 2 pounds, you could cut back to 1,400 calories a day and burn 400 more calories through exercise. It's really just a matter of individual choice, goals, and lifestyle.

Review the Calorie Deficit Chart below to see how many calories must be burned to lose up to 2 pounds per week. Your personal weekly calorie deficit will include a combination of calories you cut from your diet and calories you'll burn through exercise.

Calorie Deficit Chart

Weekly Weight Loss	Daily Calorie Deficit	Weekly Calorie Deficit
½ pound	250 calories per day	1,750 calories per week
1 pound	500 calories per day	3,500 calories per week
1 ½ pounds	750 calories per day	5,250 calories per week
2 pounds	1,000 calories per day	7,000 calories per week

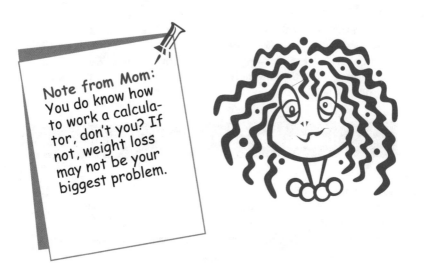

Note from Mom: You do know how to work a calculator, don't you? If not, weight loss may not be your biggest problem.

The steps that follow will walk you through the process of creating your own personal calorie deficit based on your weight loss goals. This might be a good time to grab your calculator!

In order to design an eating plan that will be most effective in helping you achieve your nutrition and weight loss goals, you'll need to create a daily calorie budget estimate that you can follow. To do this, you'll need to multiply the number for your "activity level" in the chart below by your current weight to determine how many calories you need a day to maintain your weight.

Use the chart below to determine the activity level that best describes your lifestyle. When selecting your activity level, only consider your daily routine, not your additional exercise sessions—that will happen in Step 2.

Activity Level Guide

Sedentary	Light Activity	Moderate Activity	Active
Sitting, standing, and driving most of the day	Slow walking, light gardening, light housework, but sitting quite a bit during the day	Lots of walking during the day and moderate activity over several hours most days	Very active lifestyle and/or occupation like manual labor, dancer, or very active sports played over most hours of most days
MULTIPLY BY	MULTIPLY BY	MULTIPLY BY	MULTIPLY BY
13	**14**	**15**	**16**

Okay, if you have determined your activity level number, you know your exact weight in pounds, and you have a sharpened pencil—you are officially ready to figure out your very own calorie budget! Just turn the page to begin!

14 X **175** = **2,450**

(Activity)   (Weight)   (Calories to maintain weight)

This example shows someone who is lightly active and currently weighs 175 pounds. To maintain this weight, you'd take in roughly 2,450 calories a day (14 x 175). If you take in more than 2,450 calories, you'd gain weight; take in less, and you'd lose weight—**it's just that simple.**

Now You Do It!

Use the formula below to create your own personal calorie budget for maintaining your current weight.

_____ X _____ = _____

Activity   Weight   Calories to maintain weight

Now you know roughly how many calories you need each day to stay at your current weight. However, if your goal is to lose weight, you'll need to set a new calorie budget. Use the formula on the next page to do so. Keep in mind that most health professionals recommend staying above 1,200 calories a day.

Daily Calorie Budget Formula
for Losing Weight
Example:

$$\underline{14} \times \underline{175} = \underline{2,450} - \underline{500 \text{ cal/day}} = \underline{1,950}$$

(Activity)   (Weight)   (CTMW*)   (Deficit to lose 1 lb.)   (New calorie budget)

* CTMW— Calories to maintain weight

At this weight and activity level, if you cut back to 1,950 calories per day, you'd lose about 1 pound per week because you'll have a calorie deficit of 3,500 per week. If you wanted to lose 2 pounds per week, you'll need to cut back to 1,450 calories per day, which would be a daily calorie deficit of 1,000 calories and a weekly deficit of 7,000.

Now You Do It!

Use the formula below to create your new calorie budget to lose 1 or 2 pounds per week.

_____ X _____ = _____ - **500 cal/day** = _____

Activity   Weight   CTMW   Deficit to lose 1 lb.   New calorie budget

_____ X _____ = _____ - **1000 cal/day** = _____

Activity   Weight   CTMW   Deficit to lose 2 lbs.   New calorie budget

Weekly calorie deficit from diet   =   _____

New daily calorie budget   =   _____

Remember, the best strategy for achieving weight loss is reducing calorie intake while burning more calories through exercise. So, just like a calorie budget for food intake is important, so too is a calorie expenditure budget! This is where you'll determine how often you'll exercise each week along with the number of calories you'll burn. To do this, you'll need to multiply the number of **calories burned per minute by the number of minutes that you exercise**—to give you the total calories burned per exercise session.

Use the chart below to determine how many calories are burned per minute for the specific type(s) of exercise you plan to engage in. Then decide how many days per week you to plan to exercise.

Calorie Expenditure Guide

Light Exercise	Moderate Exercise	Heavy Exercise
slow walking, light gardening, light housework, tennis (doubles), yoga calisthenics, stretching	brisk walking, swimming, moderate cycling, light weight-training, tennis (singles), beginners racquetball, light aerobics, snow skiing downhill	power walking, jogging, vigorous cycling, spinning, strenuous swimming, strenuous weight-training, Tae Bo, kick boxing, cross- country skiing
Burns calories per minute		
4	**7**	**10**

Okay, now that you've determined the various types of exercise that you will realistically engage in on a weekly basis, along with the numbers associated with them— your next step is to plug these numbers into the formula on the next page. This will determine your estimated weekly calorie expenditure.

Weekly Calorie Expenditure Formula

Example:

Exercise								
Brisk Walking	7 Cal/min.	X	45 Min./hour	X	3 Times/wk.	=	945 Cal/burned
Light Weights	7 Cal/min.	X	40 Min./hour	X	3 Times/wk.	=	840 Cal/burned

Total weekly calories burned   <u>1,785</u>

This scenario shows a total of 1,785 calories burned over the course of the week by engaging in 3 cardio sessions and 3 weight-training sessions—which is about 4 hours of exercise for the week. This number, coupled with the deficit from the example on the previous page of 3,500 calories, would result in an overall deficit of 5,285 calories for the week, which equals approximately a 1½ pound weight loss.

Use the formula below to create your calorie expenditure budget.

Now You Do It!

Exercise   _____ X _____ X _____ = _____
              Cal/min.   Min./hour   Times/wk.   Cal/burned

Exercise   _____ X _____ X _____ = _____
              Cal/min.   Min./hour   Times/wk.   Cal/burned

Total weekly calories burned   _____

Summary: Fill in the blanks below with the various calculations from the Calorie Budget Worksheet you just completed. These are your personal calorie deficit goals that will help you to reach your target weight!

- ◄ **Daily calorie budget for maintaining my current weight** _____
- ◄ **Daily calorie deficit from my diet to lose weight** _____
- ◄ **New daily calorie budget to lose weight** _____
- ◄ **Weekly calories burned through all exercise** _____
- ◄ **Total weekly calorie deficit from my diet and exercise** _____
- ◄ **Approximate pounds I'll lose per week** _____

Note: Determining the exact calorie deficit needed to lose weight is not an exact science. The calculations and formulas above do not take into account each individual's muscle mass, bone size, and other such factors—these are simply estimates. This is why it is so important to monitor your calorie intake and exercise very closely for the first several weeks of your plan. The monitoring process will allow you to tweak your calorie budget for the best and safest results.

Step 3: Food Group Servings Right For You

In Chapter 2, we said the simplest way to get all the nutrients you need each day is by using the Food Guide Pyramid as a general guide. We also mentioned that this guide shows a range of daily servings for each of the 5 major food groups, and that the number of servings you need from each group depends on how many calories you need in a given day.

The chart on the next page lists the number of servings for three basic calorie levels. See which level fits into your new calorie budget and use the suggested food group servings to create your new eating plan. If you are between calorie categories, estimate your servings!

Basic Calorie Levels

1,600 Calories: appropriate for children, sedentary women, and some older adults.

2,200 Calories: appropriate for most older children, teenage girls, active women, and sedentary men.

2,800 Calories: about right for teen boys, active men, and some very active women.

Food Groups	1,600	2,200	2,800
Whole grain servings	6 (max.)	9 (max.)	11 (max.)
Veggie servings	3 (min.)	5	5
Fruit servings	2 (min.)	4	5
Dairy servings	2-3	2-3	2-3
Meat/alternatives (in total ounces)	5 oz	6 oz	7 oz
Total fat (in grams)	53	73	93
Total added sugar (in grams)	24	48	48

Remember, following the recommended servings for the major food groups is not a rigid prescription, simply a general guide. However, in order for this to be helpful in staying within your calorie budget, be sure to adhere to proper portion sizes for each food group. See Cheat Sheet #5 for standard serving sizes for various types of foods.

You are now ready to take the information from this worksheet and create your Personal Makeover Plan!

This is where it all comes together. You are now ready to create an action plan for your personal makeover! This worksheet combines the information gleaned from the previous worksheets so that you can put your goals in writing for the following areas:

Lifestyle Habit Goals
Exercise Goals
Food Group Serving Goals
Calorie Deficit Goals

Seeing your goals on paper will give you a clear idea of what you are trying to accomplish, and it will allow you to visualize them more effectively. Plus, having this action plan to refer to each day will reinforce your goals and act as a friendly reminder, which will help you to stay on track!

Before you start writing your action plan fill in the blanks below to document your current stats so that you can track your progress throughout this process.

Personal Stats	Before	After
Current weight	_____	_____
Target Weight	_____	_____
Weight Loss Goal (lbs)	_____	_____

Healthy Habit Goals

Fill in the chart on the next page with your new, healthy habit goals that you identified on page 90. Then add a sentence or two on how you plan to achieve your new goals.

Example:

Meal Habits: I'll eat a healthy breakfast.
I will do the following: I'll eat a high-fiber cereal with 2 fruit servings and skim milk each morning.

New Healthy Lifestyle Goals	How I'll Achieve Them
General Habits	I will do the following
Meal Habits	I will do the following
Portion Control Habits	I will do the following
Nutrition Habits	I will do the following

Weekly Exercise Goals

Fill in the chart below with the types of exercise you will engage in each week, the estimated number of minutes for each session, and the number of times per week that you will do each exercise.

Exercise Type   **Minutes Per Session**   **Times Per Week**

_____

_____

_____

Food Group Serving Goals

Fill in the chart below with the food group servings you will incorporate into your new eating plan each day.

Food Group   **Number of daily servings**
Whole grains
Fruits/Veggies
Meat
Dairy

Calorie Deficit Goals*

Daily calorie budget for maintaining my current weight   _____

Daily calorie deficit goal from my diet to lose weight   _____

New daily calorie budget goal to lose weight   _____

Weekly calorie expenditure goal from exercise   _____

Total weekly calorie deficit from my diet and exercise   _____

Approximate pounds I will lose each week   _____

*Refer to the Summary information on page 100

Timeline for Reaching My Goals

If I follow this plan, it should take me approximately _____ weeks/months to meet my target weight safely.

The start date for my "Personal Makeover Plan" is _____

The target date to reach my goal is _____

The Commitment

I hereby promise to really try to implement this plan to the best of my ability. If I cheat, I will not beat myself up, but I will get right back on track with my new makeover plan!

X_____

This ends the Planning Phase—congratulations, you have officially "planned your work"! Now it's time to "work your plan" by using the activity sheets found in the next section. Good luck!

The Simple Nutrition ▶
Organizer

Chapter 9

Putting Your Makeover Plan Into Action

Things we'll cover in this chapter:	▸ Recap from the Planning Phase
	▸ Overview of the Activity Sheets
	▸ The Activity Sheets

So far, you have completed the Planning Phase of the program by creating your very own no-fail **Personal Makeover Plan**. You have officially "planned your work"—which means you are well on your way to making your weight loss and nutrition goals a reality. Just think, 50% of the work necessary to succeed is behind you! On that note, let's recap your prep work to date:

◂   **You've reviewed Simple Nutrition 101, and you now have the 411 on the most important points of nutrition and the habits of Highly Healthy Women.**

◂   **You've reviewed The Simple Nutrition Meal Plan and understand the importance of multi-tasking your meals by including lots of powerhouse foods in your daily diet.**

◂   **You've designed a detailed action plan that includes your new lifestyle habits, a calorie budget, and a realistic plan to burn calories through regular exercise.**

◂   **You've even made a written commitment to yourself to put this plan into action by designating an official start date along with a target date to reach your goals.**

You are now ready to begin the Implementation Phase by "working your plan." It's important to realize that your plan is a work in progress; it's a living document that you will modify as you discover what works for you and what doesn't work. Your plan is also designed to act as a friendly reminder of what you're trying to accomplish, which will help you to stay motivated and on track with your goals.

There Really Is No Free Lunch

By now, you've probably come to accept the fact that there really is no free lunch when it comes to permanent weight loss—no magic bullet, as they say. It boils down to lifestyle habits, eating well, and consistent exercise. If you want to see a positive change in your health and your body—you need to take action! And it's time to do just that—take your plan and put it into action with our easy-to-use activity sheets that are designed in a "day timer" format. We've provided activity sheets for 8 weeks because we think that's enough time to develop and tweak a plan that you can follow for life.

Overview of the Activity Sheets

Below are some tips on how to best use your activity sheets over the next 8 weeks. Take a look.

Weekly Meal and Exercise Sheet

The purpose of this activity sheet is to pre-plan your meals and exercise each day within a given week (we even have a place for daily "to-do's"). You may want to designate one day a week as your planning day. We think Sunday is a great day because with a fresh plan in hand you can hit the ground running on Monday. Plus, you'll have time to do the necessary prep work for the week (i.e., grocery shopping, chopping up fruits and vegetables, boiling eggs, and making dishes that can be eaten throughout the week). When choosing your meals, we recommend that you follow **The Simple Nutrition Meal Plan** in Section 2—these meals are all highly nutritious, calorie-controlled, and super easy to prepare. (Keep in mind that your total meal selections per day should be based on your daily calorie budget.) It's also important to anticipate when you'll be dining out, so you can allot yourself a certain number of calories for your dining-out experience, while staying within your calorie budget.

To simplify the program, we recommend not varying your meals too much day-to-day early on. For instance, you may want to eat the same breakfast and snacks each day, and perhaps only incorporate two meal options for lunch and dinner over the course of any given week. This will help you stick to the plan and to track your calories more closely. If variety is important, then choose completely different meal selections the following week.

Next, you will decide which days in that week you plan to exercise, the type of exercise you will engage in, and for how long. Having this exercise plan in writing will help you stick to your calorie expenditure goal. We know in the "real world" plans are subject to change. So don't despair if you deviate from your daily plan for some reason—you have all week to make up for it.

Weekly Grocery List Sheet

Once you complete your Weekly Meal and Exercise Planning Sheet, you'll be ready to make your grocery list for the week. This process is especially easy if you choose your meals from **The Simple Nutrition Meal Plan**, because we list each ingredient needed for all the meals. For those of you who shop often, this pre-printed weekly grocery list sheet will be a lifesaver—you'll have one central place to list all the things you need from the grocery store, rather than writing your list on scraps of paper that can easily get lost.

You will also **LOVE** our Best Brands List, strategically located with your activity sheets for easy referencing. We've done all the legwork by scouring the grocery store shelves and reading all the labels in order to find the most healthy and tasty brands that will make great substitutes for some of your favorite "unhealthy" foods. You'll quickly see that this list and your weekly grocery list sheets are smart timesaving tools—plus, they create less chance for unhealthy impulse buying!

Tip: To start your new eating plan on the right foot, you may want to give your pantry a makeover by doing a full-blown Pantry Raid (not to be confused with the ever-popular Panty Raid!). You should get rid of anything in your cupboards, fridge, and freezer that will sabotage your new, healthy eating plan. Say good-bye to things that contain trans fats, high amounts of sodium, refined grains, added sugars, artificial colors, nitrates, and lots of saturated fats. This would also be a good time to take an inventory of spices, oils, and vinegars as well as your storage containers for freezing meals.

Your Daily Journal Sheet

This activity sheet, which should be filled out each day, takes about five minutes to complete. You will quickly see that a food and exercise journal will help keep you honest! You'll be amazed at how many calories you didn't realize you were consuming—without it, you might tend to forget about that handful of M&M's or your kid's leftover lunch that you helped to polish off. By writing down your food intake and estimating your calories (see the Cheat Sheet on page 208 for tricks to easily eyeball calories), you can pinpoint where you are overconsuming calories or where you can make better low-calorie choices. At the end of each week, you can track your overall progress in the Progress Report section of your Journal to determine where you need to tweak your plan and set new goals, if need be, for the next week.

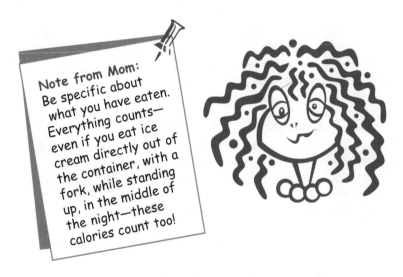

Note from Mom:
Be specific about what you have eaten. Everything counts—even if you eat ice cream directly out of the container, with a fork, while standing up, in the middle of the night—these calories count too!

When creating your Weekly Grocery List, be sure to check out our Best Brands List, located at the beginning of the activity sheets section.

But Wait, That's Not All!

In this section, you'll also find one other very important activity sheet—The Annual Health Tests by Age Group. Throughout this book, we have emphasized the importance of taking preventive measures every day for warding off chronic diseases. Equally important is early detection of diseases through regular health screenings appropriate for your age group. On this activity sheet, you'll find the list of medical tests that you should have annually for your age group, along with a place to check off each test once you've made the appointment or actually had the test done. We thought this was a great place to put this activity sheet—you'll see it every day for 8 weeks, so it will act as a reminder to make your appointments!

Let's Sum Up!

Research has shown that it takes at least 21 days to make or break a habit. By following the **Simple Nutrition For Life** plan consistently for 8 solid weeks, you are guaranteed to systematically eliminate your bad habits and replace them with healthier ones. Best of all, you will begin making significant progress on your long-term nutrition and weight loss goals, and you'll have a plan that you can follow for life!

Once you've completed your 8 weeks of activity sheets, you will have, in essence, written your own personal nutrition and weight loss plan! You will have a complete record of everything you did that worked for you—so, if you begin to backslide, you can quickly refer to your own personalized plan to help get you back on track!

So, remember—keep your nutrition and weight loss companion in a handy place because this is the central headquarters for all your nutritional and weight loss needs! Use it often, and if you leave the house, take it with you, so you can refer to it when you need it.

It's all in the details from this point forward. Ladies, start your engines...

Section 4
Activity Sheets ▶

Annual Health Tests By Age Group

Below we've listed the most common medical tests you should have by age group with a recommendation on how often. Mark off the appropriate column based on whether you have already completed the test or if you need to make an appointment (this will be friendly reminder to do so).

Ages 20-39	**How Often**	**Make Appointment/ Completed**
Physical Exam	Every 2-3 years	_____
Blood Pressure	Every 1-2 years	_____
Vision	Every 2-3 years	_____
Pap Test	Annually	_____
Breast Self-Exam	Monthly	_____
Professional Breast Exam	Annually	_____
Skin Cancer Screening	Annually	_____
Skin Self-Inspection	Monthly	_____
Cholesterol Blood Test	Every 3-5 years	_____
Dental Exam	Every 1-2 years	_____
Tetanus-Diphtheria	Every 10 years	_____

Ages 40-49	**How Often**	**Make Appointment/ Completed**
Physical Exam	Every 2-3 years	_____
Blood Pressure	Every 1-2 years	_____
Vision	Every 2-3 years	_____
Pap Test	Annually	_____
Breast Self-Exam	Monthly	_____
Professional Breast Exam	Annually	_____
Skin Cancer Screening	Annually	_____
Skin Self-Inspection	Monthly	_____
Cholesterol Blood Test	Every 3-5 years	_____
Dental Exam	Every 1-2 years	_____
Tetanus-Diphtheria	Every 10 years	_____
Mammogram	Annually	_____
Diabetes Screening	Every 3 years	_____
Digital Rectal Exam	Annually	_____

Ages 50 & Older	How Often	Make Appointment/ Completed
Physical Exam	Every 2-3 years	_____
Blood Pressure	Every 1-2 years	_____
Vision	Every 2-3 years	_____
Pap Test	Annually	_____
Breast Self-Exam	Monthly	_____
Professional Breast Exam	Annually	_____
Skin Cancer Screening	Annually	_____
Skin Self-Inspection	Monthly	_____
Cholesterol Blood Test	Every 3-5 years	_____
Dental Exam	Every 1-2 years	_____
Tetanus-Diphtheria	Every 10 years	_____
Mammogram	Annually	_____
Diabetes Screening	Every 3 years	_____
Digital Rectal Exam	Annually	_____
Glaucoma Screening	Every 2-3 years	_____
Sigmoidoscopy	Every 3-5 years	_____
Stool Blood Test	Annually	_____
Colonoscopy	Every 10 years	_____

It is important to note that these tests apply only if you are healthy and do not have symptoms of illnesses; please check with your physician otherwise. If you have an increased risk of a particular illness, testing may need to be done sooner and more often.

Tip: Be sure to take a multivitamin every day as an added insurance policy for good health!

Good nutrition and weight loss begin in the grocery store. Preparing a grocery list before you go shopping is essential in helping you to stock your pantry with healthy food choices. However, knowing which brands to buy is also very important—it can make or break your nutritional bank! You've already learned that many food manufacturers use label trickery to insinuate that their brands are healthy, when in reality many of them have hidden trans fats and high amounts of sodium, preservatives, and artificial flavorings. Take trans fats for instance. If you took an inventory of the foods that are couched as "healthy" in your kitchen, you'd probably find that trans fats (partially hydrogenated oils) are in most of the regular store brands that you buy for cereals, crackers, snack foods, and frozen meals—it's even in your coffee creamer!

In Chapter 4, we gave you plenty of tips on how to spot these imposters, but now we want to take that a step further by providing you with our list of best brands. We created our list by scouring the grocery store shelves and reading all the labels in order to find the healthiest brands that are tasty and available in most grocery stores. We chose our list of best brands based on the following merits. They must:

- Contain no trans fats.
- Contain few preservatives.
- Contain no nitrates.
- Be low in saturated fats.
- Contain few artificial flavorings.
- Be very tasty!

Some Tips For "Best Brand" Shopping

Tip #1

All varieties of the same brand are not created equal! For instance, a particular brand of canned soups may have a few varieties that are low in sodium and trans fat free, while other varieties within that same brand are packed with these evildoer ingredients. For this reason, in some cases, we list only specific varieties within a certain brand to ensure that you have access to the healthiest choices.

Tip #2

There are plenty of regular store brands that made our Best Brands List; however, many of the packaged brands will be found in the health food aisle of your grocery store and in the frozen food section—so be sure to travel down those aisles when you shop! And if you're lucky enough to live close to a health food store (i.e., Whole Foods Market), you'll find a wider selection of healthy brands.

Tip #3

Buying organic packaged brands usually ensures that you're not accidentally consuming trans fats or other additives—but it's still important to read labels because some are better than others!

Tip #4

Remember, we don't promote complete abstinence from junk food, mainly because it's unrealistic, it's too inflexible, and frankly, it's no fun! Instead, we promote moderation and making better brand choices. Once you start buying foods from our Best Brands List, you'll see that you can still enjoy your favorite foods and eat healthy at the same time!

Happy Shopping!

These varieties and brands have met our approval in terms of ingredients and taste. Our absolute favorites are in purple, these are must-have's in our book!

Cereals

General Mills Fiber One*
Barbara's Bakery Cinnamon Puffins (kids' favorite)
Kellogg's All-Bran
Kellogg's Complete Wheat Bran Flakes
Kashi Good Friends
Arrowhead Mills (all varieties)
Kashi Go Lean Crunch
Uncle Sam Cereal
Post Grape-Nuts
General Mills Multi-Bran Chex

The cereals on our list contain whole grains, have a minimum of 5 grams of fiber, no trans fats, and low amounts of sugar and sodium.

*Fiber One has 14 grams of fiber per serving—that's more than 50% of your fiber needs for the day!

Breads

StoneHearth 100% Whole Wheat
Arnold Stoneground 100% Whole Wheat
Cobblestone Mill 100% Whole Wheat
Pepperidge Farm Natural Whole Grain (9 Grain and Crunchy Grains)
Nature's Own 100% Whole Wheat
Food For Life: Ezekiel 4:9 Whole Wheat (in frozen food section)
Earth Grains Cinnamon Raisin Bagels
Toufayan Whole Wheat Pita
Goya Corn Tortillas
Lifestream Flax Plus Waffles

The breads on our list contain 100% whole grains, have a minimum of 2 grams of fiber per serving, and no trans fats.

Crackers

Kashi TLC (7-Grain and Cheddar)
Kavli Hearty Thick Crispbread
Wasa Hearty Rye Original Crispbread
Barbara's Bakery Wheatines

Unfortunately, there aren't many healthy and tasty choices when it comes to trans fat free crackers, but the Kashi TLC brand fills the void in a big way!

Chips

Tostitos Blue Corn Chips
Snyder's of Hanover Eat Smart Corn-tillas
Garden of Eatin' Tortilla Chips (all flavors)
Bearitos Tortilla Chips
Kettle Chips Potato Chips (all flavors)
Guiltless Gourmet Corn Chips
Good Health Veggie Stix
Gen Soy Soy Crips
Snyder's of Hanover Organic Pretzels

Pasta/Rice

Hodgson Mill Whole Wheat Pasta (spaghetti, spinach spaghetti & bow tie)
Annie's Whole Wheat Shells Cheddar
De Cecco Whole Wheat Linguine
Ancient Harvest Quinoa Pasta
DeBoles Whole Wheat Spaghetti
Uncle Ben's Instant Brown Rice
Fantastic Whole Wheat Couscous
Fantastic Brown Basmati Rice
Success 10-Minute Brown Rice

Soups/Sauces/Dressings/Other

Health Valley Vegetable Soup (low sodium)
Health Valley Chili (no salt added)
Health Valley Lentil & Carrot (low sodium)
Progresso Lentil Soup
Bertolli Tomato & Basil Pasta Sauce
Classico Tomato & Basil Pasta Sauce
Tostitos All Natural Salsa
Wish-Bone Balsamic Vinaigrette
Nasoya Dressings (all flavors)
Newman's Own Light Raspberry and Walnut Dressing
Green Giant Whole Kernel Sweet Corn (50% less sodium)
Stokely's Cut Green Beans (no salt added)
Del Monte Pear Halves (extra light syrup)
Lipton 100% Natural Green Tea
Del Monte Sliced Pineapple (packed in its own juice)

Regular store brands that offer low or reduced sodium and sugar can be hard to find—so if you do find them, be sure to stock up!

Meat/Meat Substitutes

Gorton's Frozen Salmon
Hormel Pork Tenderloin
StarKist Albacore Tuna (packed in water)
Contessa Frozen Cooked Shrimp
Contessa Stir Fry Shrimp or Chicken
Boar's Head Oven Roasted Sliced Turkey
Smucker's Natural Peanut Butter
GardenBurgers (all types)
Morningstar Farms Veggie Burgers (all kinds)
Light Smart Soy Dogs
Athenos Hummus (all types)
Yves Veggie Cuisine (all types)
Amy's Frozen Meals and TV Dinners
Cascadian Farm Veggie Bowls (all types)

Most regular store brand frozen meals contain trans fats and high amounts of sodium. The brands we listed above are better choices. However, even these healthier brands contain high amounts of sodium. Try to limit your intake of even these healthy frozen meals.

Fruits/Veggies

Green Giant Frozen Veggies
Cascadian Farm Organic Frozen Fruits
Minute Maid Frozen Orange Juice
Earthbound Farm Organic Baby Spinach
Any fresh fruit or veggie by any brand!

Dairy

Dannon Lowfat Yogurt (plain/fruit)
Stoneyfield Farm Lowfat Yogurt
Silk Soy French Vanilla Creamer
Silk Soy Milk
Jarlsberg Lite Swiss Cheese
Kraft Reduced Fat Cheddar Cheese
Cabot Vermont Cheddar Cheese 50% Light
Horizons Organic String Cheese
Smart Beat Trans Fat Free Light Margarine
Smart Balance Spread
Egg-Land's Best (110 mg Omega3)
Egg Beaters

Desserts/Snacks

The "Skinny Cow" Silhouette Fudge Bars
Edy's Whole Fruit Fruit Bars
Starbucks Frappuccino Bar
Nature Valley Granola Bars (all flavors)
Luna Bars (all flavors)
Barbara's Bakery Multigrain Cereal Bars (all flavors)
Newman's Own Alphabet Cookies (Cinnamon)
Newman-O's
Barbara's Bakery Organic Go Go Graham Crackers
Barbara's Bakery Crisp Cookies Chocolate Chip
Mi-Del GingerSnaps
Health Valley Healthy Chips Double Chocolate Cookies

Week #_____   _____ **to** _____

List the meals you plan to have each day over the next week along with the
estimated calories for each meal. Be sure to document when you will be dining out.

Breakfast	Lunch	Dinner	Snacks
		MONDAY	
Cal.	Cal.	Cal.	Cal.

Breakfast	Lunch	Dinner	Snacks
		TUESDAY	
Cal.	Cal.	Cal.	Cal.

Breakfast	Lunch	Dinner	Snacks
		WEDNESDAY	
Cal.	Cal.	Cal.	Cal.

Breakfast	Lunch	Dinner	Snacks
		THURSDAY	
Cal.	Cal.	Cal.	Cal.

Weekday To-do's	

Daily Healthy Habit Reminders

Make doctor appointments.
Stock fridge with healthy foods.
Pack snacks to go.
Drink 8 glasses of water daily.
Exercise on designated days.
Write in your journal every day.

Review action plan daily.
Prepare meals in advance.
Practice portion control.
Start a green tea habit.
Reward yourself.
Take a multivitamin every day.

Breakfast	Lunch	Dinner	Snacks
		FRIDAY	
Cal.	Cal.	Cal.	Cal.

Breakfast	Lunch	Dinner	Snacks
		SATURDAY	
Cal.	Cal.	Cal.	Cal.

Breakfast	Lunch	Dinner	Snacks
		SUNDAY	
Cal.	Cal.	Cal.	Cal.

Weekend To-do's

List the types of exercises you will do this week and place an x on the day you plan to do them.

Exercise	Mon	Tue	Wed	Thur	Fri	Sat	Sun

Weekly Grocery List Sheets

Week # _____   _____ to _____ Total Spent $_____

Whole Grains	Produce

Dairy	Meat/Poultry/Fish/Deli

Condiments	Frozen

Canned Goods	Packaged Goods

Cleaning/Paper Supplies	Miscellaneous

Avoid:	Include:
Saturated fats	**Good fats** (olive oil, avocado, etc.)
Trans fats (partially hydrogenated oils)	**Low-fat dairy and meats**
Palm kernel oil, lard, shortening	**High-fiber cereals** (min 5 grams)
Refined grains	**100% whole-grain bread**
Artificial flavorings	**100% fruit juice**
Olestra	**Foods with no preservatives**
Nitrates	**Low-sodium canned goods**
Hidden added sugars	**Flavored green tea**
Pastries, sodas, and sugary cereals	**Raw nuts**
Hidden sodium	**Legumes**
Full -fat meats	**Beans and peas**
Full -fat dairy	**Deep-colored fruits and veggies**

Daily Journal Sheets

Week #_____   _____ **to** _____

List everything you eat and drink each day. Be sure to track calories and food group servings too.

Breakfast	Lunch	Dinner	Snacks	Other
		MONDAY		**Grain** _____ **Fruit** _____ **Veg** _____ **Meat** _____ **Dairy** _____
Cal.	Cal.	Cal.	Cal.	Tot. Cal.

Breakfast	Lunch	Dinner	Snacks	Other
		TUESDAY		**Grain** _____ **Fruit** _____ **Veg** _____ **Meat** _____ **Dairy** _____
Cal.	Cal.	Cal.	Cal.	Tot. Cal.

Breakfast	Lunch	Dinner	Snacks	Other
				Grain _____ **Fruit** _____ **Veg** _____ **Meat** _____ **Dairy** _____
Cal.	Cal.	Cal.	Cal.	Tot.Cal.

WEDNESDAY

Breakfast	Lunch	Dinner	Snacks	Other
				Grain _____ **Fruit** _____ **Veg** _____ **Meat** _____ **Dairy** _____
Cal.	Cal.	Cal.	Cal.	Tot.Cal.

THURSDAY

Breakfast	Lunch	Dinner	Snacks	Other
				Grain _____
				Fruit _____
		FRIDAY		Veg _____
				Meat _____
				Dairy _____
Cal.	Cal.	Cal.	Cal.	Tot. Cal.

Breakfast	Lunch	Dinner	Snacks	Other
				Grain _____
				Fruit _____
		SATURDAY		Veg _____
				Meat _____
				Dairy _____
Cal.	Cal.	Cal.	Cal.	Tot. Cal.

Breakfast	Lunch	Dinner	Snacks	Other
				Grain _____
				Fruit _____
				Veg _____
				Meat _____
		SUNDAY		Dairy _____
Cal.	Cal.	Cal.	Cal.	Tot. Cal.

Exercise	Day of Week	Hrs/Min.	Calories Burned

Weekly Progress Report   <u>Goal</u>   <u>Actual</u>

Total calories consumed this week   _____   _____
Total calories burned this week   _____   _____
Total weight lost this week   _____   _____

Things I'll do next week to improve: _____

_____

_____

Weekly Meal and Exercise Planning Sheets

Week #_____   _____ **to** _____

List the meals you plan to have each day over the next week along with the
estimated calories for each meal. Be sure to document when you will be dining out.

Breakfast	Lunch	Dinner	Snacks
		MONDAY	
Cal.	Cal.	Cal.	Cal.

Breakfast	Lunch	Dinner	Snacks
		TUESDAY	
Cal.	Cal.	Cal.	Cal.

Breakfast	Lunch	Dinner	Snacks
		WEDNESDAY	
Cal.	Cal.	Cal.	Cal.

Breakfast	Lunch	Dinner	Snacks
		THURSDAY	
Cal.	Cal.	Cal.	Cal.

Weekday To-do's	

Daily Healthy Habit Reminders

Make doctor appointments.
Stock fridge with healthy foods.
Pack snacks to go.
Drink 8 glasses of water daily.
Exercise on designated days.
Write in your journal every day.

Review action plan daily.
Prepare meals in advance.
Practice portion control.
Start a green tea habit.
Reward yourself.
Take a multivitamin every day.

Breakfast	Lunch	Dinner	Snacks
		FRIDAY	
Cal.	Cal.	Cal.	Cal.

Breakfast	Lunch	Dinner	Snacks
		SATURDAY	
Cal.	Cal.	Cal.	Cal.

Breakfast	Lunch	Dinner	Snacks

SUNDAY

Cal.	Cal.	Cal.	Cal.

Weekend To-do's	

List the types of exercises you will do this week and place an x on the day you plan to do them.

Exercise	Mon	Tue	Wed	Thur	Fri	Sat	Sun

Weekly Grocery List Sheets

Week # _____   _____ to _____ Total Spent $_____

Whole Grains	Produce

Dairy	Meat/Poultry/Fish/Deli

Condiments	Frozen

Canned Goods	Packaged Goods

Cleaning/Paper Supplies	Miscellaneous

Avoid:	Include:
Saturated fats	Good fats (olive oil, avocado, etc.)
Trans fats (partially hydrogenated oils)	Low-fat dairy and meats
Palm kernel oil, lard, shortening	High-fiber cereals (min. 5 grams)
Refined grains	100% whole-grain bread
Artificial flavorings	100% fruit juice
Olestra	Foods with no preservatives
Nitrates	Low-sodium canned goods
Hidden added sugars	Flavored green tea
Pastries, sodas, and sugary cereals	Raw nuts
Hidden sodium	Legumes
Full-fat meats	Beans and peas
Full-fat dairy	Deep-colored fruits and veggies

Daily Journal Sheets

Week #_____   _____ **to** _____

List everything you eat and drink each day. Be sure to track calories and food group servings too.

Breakfast	Lunch	Dinner	Snacks	Other
		MONDAY		**Grain** _____ **Fruit** _____ **Veg** _____ **Meat** _____ **Dairy** _____
Cal.	Cal.	Cal.	Cal.	Tot. Cal.

Breakfast	Lunch	Dinner	Snacks	Other
		TUESDAY		**Grain** _____ **Fruit** _____ **Veg** _____ **Meat** _____ **Dairy** _____
Cal.	Cal.	Cal.	Cal.	Tot. Cal.

Breakfast	Lunch	Dinner	Snacks	Other
				Grain _____
				Fruit _____
				Veg _____
				Meat _____
		WEDNESDAY		**Dairy** _____
Cal.	Cal.	Cal.	Cal.	Tot. Cal.

Breakfast	Lunch	Dinner	Snacks	Other
				Grain _____
				Fruit _____
				Veg _____
				Meat _____
		THURSDAY		**Dairy** _____
Cal.	Cal.	Cal.	Cal.	Tot. Cal.

Breakfast	Lunch	Dinner	Snacks	Other
				Grain _____
				Fruit _____
				Veg _____
				Meat _____
			FRIDAY	**Dairy** _____
Cal.	Cal.	Cal.	Cal.	Tot.Cal.

Breakfast	Lunch	Dinner	Snacks	Other
				Grain _____
				Fruit _____
				Veg _____
				Meat _____
		SATURDAY		**Dairy** _____
Cal.	Cal.	Cal.	Cal.	Tot.Cal.

Breakfast	Lunch	Dinner	Snacks	Other
				Grain _____
				Fruit _____
				Veg _____
				Meat _____
				Dairy _____
		SUNDAY		
Cal.	Cal.	Cal.	Cal.	Tot. Cal.

Exercise	Day of Week	Hrs/Min.	Calories Burned

Weekly Progress Report	**Goal**	**Actual**
Total calories consumed this week	_____	_____
Total calories burned this week	_____	_____
Total weight lost this week	_____	_____

Things I'll do next week to improve: _____

_____

_____

Week #_____   _____ **to** _____

List the meals you plan to have each day over the next week along with the
estimated calories for each meal. Be sure to document when you will be dining out.

Breakfast	Lunch	Dinner	Snacks
		MONDAY	
Cal.	Cal.	Cal.	Cal.
Breakfast	Lunch	Dinner	Snacks
		TUESDAY	
Cal.	Cal.	Cal.	Cal.

Breakfast	Lunch	Dinner	Snacks
		WEDNESDAY	
Cal.	Cal.	Cal.	Cal.

Breakfast	Lunch	Dinner	Snacks
		THURSDAY	
Cal.	Cal.	Cal.	Cal.

Weekday To-do's	

Daily Healthy Habit Reminders

Make doctor appointments.
Stock fridge with healthy foods.
Pack snacks to go.
Drink 8 glasses of water daily.
Exercise on designated days.
Write in your journal every day.

Review action plan daily.
Prepare meals in advance.
Practice portion control.
Start a green tea habit.
Reward yourself.
Take a multivitamin every day.

Breakfast	Lunch	Dinner	Snacks
		FRIDAY	
Cal.	Cal.	Cal.	Cal.

Breakfast	Lunch	Dinner	Snacks
		SATURDAY	
Cal.	Cal.	Cal.	Cal.

Breakfast	Lunch	Dinner	Snacks
		SUNDAY	
Cal.	Cal.	Cal.	Cal.

Weekend To-do's

List the types of exercises you will do this week and place an x on the day you plan to do them.

Exercise	Mon	Tue	Wed	Thur	Fri	Sat	Sun

Weekly Grocery List Sheets

Week # _____   _____ to _____ Total Spent $_____

Whole Grains	Produce

Dairy	Meat/Poultry/Fish/Deli

Condiments	Frozen

Canned Goods	Packaged Goods

Cleaning/Paper Supplies	Miscellaneous

Avoid:	Include:
Saturated fats	Good fats (olive oil, avocado, etc.)
Trans fats (partially hydrogenated oils)	Low-fat dairy and meats
Palm kernel oil, lard, shortening	High-fiber cereals (min. 5 grams)
Refined grains	100% whole-grain bread
Artificial flavorings	100% fruit juice
Olestra	Foods with no preservatives
Nitrates	Low-sodium canned goods
Hidden added sugars	Flavored green tea
Pastries, sodas, and sugary cereals	Raw nuts
Hidden sodium	Legumes
Full-fat meats	Beans and peas
Full-fat dairy	Deep-colored fruits and veggies

Daily Journal Sheets

Week #_____   _____ **to** _____

List everything you eat and drink each day. Be sure to track calories and food group servings too.

Breakfast	Lunch	Dinner	Snacks	Other
				Grain _____ **Fruit** _____ **Veg** _____ **Meat** _____ **Dairy** _____
Cal.	Cal.	Cal.	Cal.	Tot. Cal.
Breakfast	**Lunch**	**Dinner**	**Snacks**	**Other**
				Grain _____ **Fruit** _____ **Veg** _____ **Meat** _____ **Dairy** _____
Cal.	Cal.	Cal.	Cal.	Tot. Cal.

MONDAY

TUESDAY

Breakfast	Lunch	Dinner	Snacks	Other
				Grain _____
				Fruit _____
				Veg _____
				Meat _____
		WEDNESDAY		Dairy _____
Cal.	Cal.	Cal.	Cal.	Tot. Cal.

Breakfast	Lunch	Dinner	Snacks	Other
				Grain _____
				Fruit _____
				Veg _____
				Meat _____
		THURSDAY		Dairy _____
Cal.	Cal.	Cal.	Cal.	Tot. Cal.

Breakfast	Lunch	Dinner	Snacks	Other
				Grain _____
				Fruit _____
				Veg _____
				Meat _____
		FRIDAY		**Dairy** _____
Cal.	Cal.	Cal.	Cal.	Tot. Cal.

Breakfast	Lunch	Dinner	Snacks	Other
				Grain _____
				Fruit _____
				Veg _____
				Meat _____
		SATURDAY		**Dairy** _____
Cal.	Cal.	Cal.	Cal.	Tot. Cal.

Breakfast	Lunch	Dinner	Snacks	Other
				Grain _____
				Fruit _____
				Veg _____
				Meat _____
				Dairy _____
Cal.	Cal.	Cal.	Cal.	Tot. Cal.

SUNDAY

Exercise	Day of Week	Hrs/Min.	Calories Burned

Weekly Progress Report	**Goal**	**Actual**

Total calories consumed this week _____ _____
Total calories burned this week _____ _____
Total weight lost this week _____ _____

Things I'll do next week to improve: _____

_____

_____

Week #_____   _____ **to** _____

List the meals you plan to have each day over the next week along with the estimated calories for each meal. Be sure to document when you will be dining out.

Breakfast	Lunch	Dinner	Snacks
	MONDAY		
Cal.	Cal.	Cal.	Cal.

Breakfast	Lunch	Dinner	Snacks
	TUESDAY		
Cal.	Cal.	Cal.	Cal.

Breakfast	Lunch	Dinner	Snacks
		WEDNESDAY	
Cal.	Cal.	Cal.	Cal.

Breakfast	Lunch	Dinner	Snacks
		THURSDAY	
Cal.	Cal.	Cal.	Cal.

Weekday To-do's	

Daily Healthy Habit Reminders

Make doctor appointments.
Stock fridge with healthy foods.
Pack snacks to go.
Drink 8 glasses of water daily.
Exercise on designated days.
Write in your journal every day.

Review action plan daily.
Prepare meals in advance.
Practice portion control.
Start a green tea habit.
Reward yourself.
Take a multivitamin every day.

Breakfast	Lunch	Dinner	Snacks
		FRIDAY	
Cal.	Cal.	Cal.	Cal.

Breakfast	Lunch	Dinner	Snacks
		SATURDAY	
Cal.	Cal.	Cal.	Cal.

Breakfast	Lunch	Dinner	Snacks
		SUNDAY	
Cal.	Cal.	Cal.	Cal.

Weekend To-do's	

List the types of exercises you will do this week and place an x on the day you plan to do them.

Exercise	Mon	Tue	Wed	Thur	Fri	Sat	Sun

Weekly Grocery List Sheets

Week # _____   _____ to _____   Total Spent $_____

Whole Grains	Produce

Dairy	Meat/Poultry/Fish/Deli

Condiments	Frozen

Canned Goods	Packaged Goods

Cleaning/Paper Supplies	Miscellaneous

Avoid:	Include:
Saturated fats	Good fats (olive oil, avocado, etc.)
Trans fats (partially hydrogenated oils)	Low-fat dairy and meats
Palm kernel oil, lard, shortening	High-fiber cereals (min. 5 grams)
Refined grains	100% whole-grain bread
Artificial flavorings	100% fruit juice
Olestra	Foods with no preservatives
Nitrates	Low-sodium canned goods
Hidden added sugars	Flavored green tea
Pastries, sodas, and sugary cereals	Raw nuts
Hidden sodium	Legumes
Full-fat meats	Beans and peas
Full-fat dairy	Deep-colored fruits and veggies

Week #_____   _____ **to** _____

List everything you eat and drink each day. Be sure to track calories and food group servings too.

Breakfast	Lunch	Dinner	Snacks	Other
		MONDAY		**Grain** _____ **Fruit** _____ **Veg** _____ **Meat** _____ **Dairy** _____
Cal.	Cal.	Cal.	Cal.	Tot. Cal.

Breakfast	Lunch	Dinner	Snacks	Other
		TUESDAY		**Grain** _____ **Fruit** _____ **Veg** _____ **Meat** _____ **Dairy** _____
Cal.	Cal.	Cal.	Cal.	Tot. Cal.

Breakfast	Lunch	Dinner	Snacks	Other
				Grain _____
				Fruit _____
				Veg _____
				Meat _____
				Dairy _____
		WEDNESDAY		
Cal.	Cal.	Cal.	Cal.	Tot. Cal.

Breakfast	Lunch	Dinner	Snacks	Other
				Grain _____
				Fruit _____
				Veg _____
				Meat _____
				Dairy _____
		THURSDAY		
Cal.	Cal.	Cal.	Cal.	Tot. Cal.

Breakfast	Lunch	Dinner	Snacks	Other
				Grain _____ **Fruit** _____ **Veg** _____ **Meat** _____ **Dairy** _____
Cal.	Cal.	Cal.	Cal.	Tot. Cal.

FRIDAY

Breakfast	Lunch	Dinner	Snacks	Other
				Grain _____ **Fruit** _____ **Veg** _____ **Meat** _____ **Dairy** _____
Cal.	Cal.	Cal.	Cal.	Tot. Cal.

SATURDAY

Breakfast	Lunch	Dinner	Snacks	Other
				Grain _____
				Fruit _____
				Veg _____
				Meat _____
		SUNDAY		Dairy _____
Cal.	Cal.	Cal.	Cal.	Tot. Cal.

Exercise	Day of Week	Hrs/Min.	Calories Burned

Weekly Progress Report   Goal   Actual

Total calories consumed this week   _____   _____
Total calories burned this week   _____   _____
Total weight lost this week   _____   _____

Things I'll do next week to improve: _____

_____

_____

Weekly Meal and Exercise Planning Sheets

Week #_____   _____ **to** _____

List the meals you plan to have each day over the next week along with the estimated calories for each meal. Be sure to document when you will be dining out.

Breakfast	Lunch	Dinner	Snacks
		MONDAY	
Cal.	Cal.	Cal.	Cal.
Breakfast	**Lunch**	**Dinner**	**Snacks**
		TUESDAY	
Cal.	Cal.	Cal.	Cal.

Breakfast	Lunch	Dinner	Snacks
		WEDNESDAY	
Cal.	Cal.	Cal.	Cal.

Breakfast	Lunch	Dinner	Snacks
		THURSDAY	
Cal.	Cal.	Cal.	Cal.

Weekday To-do's	

Daily Healthy Habit Reminders

Make doctor appointments.
Stock fridge with healthy foods.
Pack snacks to go.
Drink 8 glasses of water daily.
Exercise on designated days.
Write in your journal every day.

Review action plan daily.
Prepare meals in advance.
Practice portion control.
Start a green tea habit.
Reward yourself.
Take a multi vitamin every day.

Breakfast	Lunch	Dinner	Snacks
		FRIDAY	
Cal.	Cal.	Cal.	Cal.

Breakfast	Lunch	Dinner	Snacks
		SATURDAY	
Cal.	Cal.	Cal.	Cal.

Breakfast	Lunch	Dinner	Snacks
		SUNDAY	
Cal.	Cal.	Cal.	Cal.

Weekend To-do's	

List the types of exercises you will do this week and place an x on the day you plan to do them.

Exercise	Mon	Tue	Wed	Thur	Fri	Sat	Sun

Weekly Grocery List Sheets

Week # _____   ____ to ____ Total Spent $_____

Whole Grains	Produce

Dairy	Meat/Poultry/Fish/Deli

Condiments	Frozen

Canned Goods	Packaged Goods

Cleaning/Paper Supplies	Miscellaneous

Avoid:	Include:
Saturated fats	Good fats (olive oil, avocado, etc.)
Trans fats (partially hydrogenated oils)	Low-fat dairy and meats
Palm kernel oil, lard, shortening	High-fiber cereals (min. 5 grams)
Refined grains	100% whole-grain bread
Artificial flavorings	100% fruit juice
Olestra	Foods with no preservatives
Nitrates	Low-sodium canned goods
Hidden added sugars	Flavored green tea
Pastries, sodas, and sugary cereals	Raw nuts
Hidden sodium	Legumes
Full-fat meats	Beans and peas
Full-fat dairy	Deep-colored fruits and veggies

Daily Journal Sheets

Week #_____   _____ **to** _____

List everything you eat and drink each day. Be sure to track calories and food group servings too.

Breakfast	Lunch	Dinner	Snacks	Other
		MONDAY		**Grain** _____ **Fruit** _____ **Veg** _____ **Meat** _____ **Dairy** _____
Cal.	Cal.	Cal.	Cal.	Tot. Cal.

Breakfast	Lunch	Dinner	Snacks	Other
		TUESDAY		**Grain** _____ **Fruit** _____ **Veg** _____ **Meat** _____ **Dairy** _____
Cal.	Cal.	Cal.	Cal.	Tot. Cal.

Breakfast	Lunch	Dinner	Snacks	Other
				Grain _____
				Fruit _____
				Veg _____
				Meat _____
			WEDNESDAY	Dairy _____
Cal.	Cal.	Cal.	Cal.	Tot. Cal.

Breakfast	Lunch	Dinner	Snacks	Other
				Grain _____
				Fruit _____
				Veg _____
				Meat _____
			THURSDAY	Dairy _____
Cal.	Cal.	Cal.	Cal.	Tot. Cal.

Breakfast	Lunch	Dinner	Snacks	Other
		FRIDAY		Grain _____ Fruit _____ Veg _____ Meat _____ Dairy _____
Cal.	Cal.	Cal.	Cal.	Tot. Cal.

Breakfast	Lunch	Dinner	Snacks	Other
		SATURDAY		Grain _____ Fruit _____ Veg _____ Meat _____ Dairy _____
Cal.	Cal.	Cal.	Cal.	Tot. Cal.

Breakfast	Lunch	Dinner	Snacks	Other
				Grain _____
				Fruit _____
				Veg _____
				Meat _____
				Dairy _____
		SUNDAY		
Cal.	Cal.	Cal.	Cal.	Tot. Cal.

Exercise	Day of Week	Hrs/Min.	Calories Burned

Weekly Progress Report   Goal   Actual

Total calories consumed this week   _____   _____

Total calories burned this week   _____   _____

Total weight lost this week   _____   _____

Things I'll do next week to improve: _____

_____

_____

Week #_____   _____ **to** _____

List the meals you plan to have each day over the next week along with the
estimated calories for each meal. Be sure to document when you will be dining out.

Breakfast	Lunch	Dinner	Snacks
		MONDAY	
Cal.	Cal.	Cal.	Cal.
Breakfast	Lunch	Dinner	Snacks
		TUESDAY	
Cal.	Cal.	Cal.	Cal.

Breakfast	Lunch	Dinner	Snacks
		WEDNESDAY	
Cal.	Cal.	Cal.	Cal.

Breakfast	Lunch	Dinner	Snacks
		THURSDAY	
Cal.	Cal.	Cal.	Cal.

Weekday To-do's	

Daily Healthy Habit Reminders

Make doctor appointments.
Stock fridge with healthy foods.
Pack snacks to go.
Drink 8 glasses of water daily.
Exercise on designated days.
Write in your journal every day.

Review action plan daily.
Prepare meals in advance.
Practice portion control.
Start a green tea habit.
Reward yourself.
Take a multivitamin every day.

Breakfast	Lunch	Dinner	Snacks
		FRIDAY	
Cal.	Cal.	Cal.	Cal.

Breakfast	Lunch	Dinner	Snacks
		SATURDAY	
Cal.	Cal.	Cal.	Cal.

Breakfast	Lunch	Dinner	Snacks
		SUNDAY	
Cal.	Cal.	Cal.	Cal.

Weekend To-do's	

List the types of exercises you will do this week and place an x on the day you plan to do them.

Exercise	Mon	Tue	Wed	Thur	Fri	Sat	Sun

Weekly Grocery List Sheets

Week # _____   _____ to _____   Total Spent $_____

Whole Grains

Produce

Dairy

Meat/Poultry/Fish/Deli

Condiments

Frozen

Canned Goods	Packaged Goods

Cleaning/Paper Supplies	Miscellaneous

Avoid:	Include:
Saturated fats	Good fats (olive oil, avocado, etc.)
Trans fats (partially hydrogenated oils)	Low-fat dairy and meats
Palm kernel oil, lard, shortening	High-fiber cereals (min. 5 grams)
Refined grains	100% whole-grain bread
Artificial flavorings	100% fruit juice
Olestra	Foods with no preservatives
Nitrates	Low-sodium canned goods
Hidden added sugars	Flavored green tea
Pastries, sodas, and sugary cereals	Raw nuts
Hidden sodium	Legumes
Full-fat meats	Beans and peas
Full-fat dairy	Deep-colored fruits and veggies

Daily Journal Sheets

Week #_____   _____ **to** _____

List everything you eat and drink each day. Be sure to track calories and food group servings too.

Breakfast	Lunch	Dinner	Snacks	Other
		MONDAY		**Grain** _____ **Fruit** _____ **Veg** _____ **Meat** _____ **Dairy** _____
Cal.	Cal.	Cal.	Cal.	Tot. Cal.
Breakfast	Lunch	Dinner	Snacks	Other
		TUESDAY		**Grain** _____ **Fruit** _____ **Veg** _____ **Meat** _____ **Dairy** _____
Cal.	Cal.	Cal.	Cal.	Tot. Cal.

Breakfast	Lunch	Dinner	Snacks	Other
		WEDNESDAY		**Grain** _____ **Fruit** _____ **Veg** _____ **Meat** _____ **Dairy** _____
Cal.	Cal.	Cal.	Cal.	Tot. Cal.

Breakfast	Lunch	Dinner	Snacks	Other
		THURSDAY		**Grain** _____ **Fruit** _____ **Veg** _____ **Meat** _____ **Dairy** _____
Cal.	Cal.	Cal.	Cal.	Tot. Cal.

Breakfast	Lunch	Dinner	Snacks	Other
				Grain _____
				Fruit _____
				Veg _____
				Meat _____
		FRIDAY		**Dairy** _____
Cal.	Cal.	Cal.	Cal.	Tot. Cal.

Breakfast	Lunch	Dinner	Snacks	Other
				Grain _____
				Fruit _____
				Veg _____
				Meat _____
		SATURDAY		**Dairy** _____
Cal.	Cal.	Cal.	Cal.	Tot. Cal.

Breakfast	Lunch	Dinner	Snacks	Other
				Grain _____
				Fruit _____
		SUNDAY		Veg _____
				Meat _____
				Dairy _____
Cal.	Cal.	Cal.	Cal.	Tot. Cal.

Exercise	Day of Week	Hrs/Min.	Calories Burned

Weekly Progress Report	**Goal**	**Actual**
Total calories consumed this week	_____	_____
Total calories burned this week	_____	_____
Total weight lost this week	_____	_____

Things I'll do next week to improve: _____

_____

_____

Week #_____   _____ **to** _____

List the meals you plan to have each day over the next week along with the
estimated calories for each meal. Be sure to document when you will be dining out.

Breakfast	Lunch	Dinner	Snacks
		MONDAY	
Cal.	Cal.	Cal.	Cal.

Breakfast	Lunch	Dinner	Snacks
		TUESDAY	
Cal.	Cal.	Cal.	Cal.

Breakfast	Lunch	Dinner	Snacks
WEDNESDAY			
Cal.	Cal.	Cal.	Cal.

Breakfast	Lunch	Dinner	Snacks
THURSDAY			
Cal.	Cal.	Cal.	Cal.

Weekday To-do's	

Daily Healthy Habit Reminders

Make doctor appointments.
Stock fridge with healthy foods.
Pack snacks to go.
Drink 8 glasses of water daily.
Exercise on designated days.
Write in your journal every day.

Review action plan daily.
Prepare meals in advance.
Practice portion control.
Start a green tea habit.
Reward yourself.
Take a multivitamin every day.

Breakfast	Lunch	Dinner	Snacks
		FRIDAY	
Cal.	Cal.	Cal.	Cal.

Breakfast	Lunch	Dinner	Snacks
		SATURDAY	
Cal.	Cal.	Cal.	Cal.

Breakfast	Lunch	Dinner	Snacks
		SUNDAY	
Cal.	Cal.	Cal.	Cal.

Weekend To-do's	

List the types of exercises you will do this week and place an x on the day you plan to do them.

Exercise	Mon	Tue	Wed	Thur	Fri	Sat	Sun

Weekly Grocery List Sheets

Week # _____   _____ to _____ Total Spent $_____

Whole Grains	Produce

Dairy	Meat/Poultry/Fish/Deli

Condiments	Frozen

Canned Goods	Packaged Goods

Cleaning/Paper Supplies	Miscellaneous

Avoid:	Include:
Saturated fats	Good fats (olive oil, avocado, etc.)
Trans fats (partially hydrogenated oils)	Low-fat dairy and meats
Palm kernel oil, lard, shortening	High-fiber cereals (min. 5 grams)
Refined grains	100% whole-grain bread
Artificial flavorings	100% fruit juice
Olestra	Foods with no preservatives
Nitrates	Low-sodium canned goods
Hidden added sugars	Flavored green tea
Pastries, sodas, and sugary cereals	Raw nuts
Hidden sodium	Legumes
Full-fat meats	Beans and peas
Full-fat dairy	Deep-colored fruits and veggies

Daily Journal Sheets

Week #_____   _____ **to** _____

List everything you eat and drink each day. Be sure to track calories and food group servings too.

Breakfast	Lunch	Dinner	Snacks	Other
				Grain _____
				Fruit _____
				Veg _____
				Meat _____
		MONDAY		**Dairy** _____
Cal.	Cal.	Cal.	Cal.	Tot. Cal.
Breakfast	Lunch	Dinner	Snacks	Other
				Grain _____
				Fruit _____
				Veg _____
				Meat _____
		TUESDAY		**Dairy** _____
Cal.	Cal.	Cal.	Cal.	Tot. Cal.

Breakfast	Lunch	Dinner	Snacks	Other
				Grain _____
				Fruit _____
				Veg _____
				Meat _____
				Dairy _____
		WEDNESDAY		
Cal.	Cal.	Cal.	Cal.	Tot. Cal.

Breakfast	Lunch	Dinner	Snacks	Other
				Grain _____
				Fruit _____
				Veg _____
				Meat _____
				Dairy _____
		THURSDAY		
Cal.	Cal.	Cal.	Cal.	Tot. Cal.

Breakfast	Lunch	Dinner	Snacks	Other
				Grain _____
				Fruit _____
				Veg _____
				Meat _____
				Dairy _____
		FRIDAY		
Cal.	Cal.	Cal.	Cal.	Tot.Cal.

Breakfast	Lunch	Dinner	Snacks	Other
				Grain _____
				Fruit _____
				Veg _____
				Meat _____
				Dairy _____
		SATURDAY		
Cal.	Cal.	Cal.	Cal.	Tot.Cal.

Breakfast	Lunch	Dinner	Snacks	Other
				Grain _____
				Fruit _____
				Veg _____
				Meat _____
		SUNDAY		Dairy _____
Cal.	Cal.	Cal.	Cal.	Tot. Cal.

Exercise	Day of Week	Hrs/Min.	Calories Burned

Weekly Progress Report

	Goal	Actual
Total calories consumed this week	_____	_____
Total calories burned this week	_____	_____
Total weight lost this week	_____	_____

Things I'll do next week to improve: _____

_____

_____

Weekly Meal and Exercise Planning Sheets

Week #_____   _____ **to** _____

List the meals you plan to have each day over the next week along with the estimated calories for each meal. Be sure to document when you will be dining out.

Breakfast	Lunch	Dinner	Snacks
		MONDAY	
Cal.	Cal.	Cal.	Cal.
Breakfast	**Lunch**	**Dinner**	**Snacks**
		TUESDAY	
Cal.	Cal.	Cal.	Cal.

Breakfast	Lunch	Dinner	Snacks
		WEDNESDAY	
Cal.	Cal.	Cal.	Cal.

Breakfast	Lunch	Dinner	Snacks
		THURSDAY	
Cal.	Cal.	Cal.	Cal.

Weekday To-do's	

Daily Healthy Habit Reminders

Make doctor appointments.
Stock fridge with healthy foods.
Pack snacks to go.
Drink 8 glasses of water daily.
Exercise on designated days.
Write in your journal every day.

Review action plan daily.
Prepare meals in advance.
Practice portion control.
Start a green tea habit.
Reward yourself.
Take a multivitamin every day.

Breakfast	Lunch	Dinner	Snacks
		FRIDAY	
Cal.	Cal.	Cal.	Cal.

Breakfast	Lunch	Dinner	Snacks
		SATURDAY	
Cal.	Cal.	Cal.	Cal.

Breakfast	Lunch	Dinner	Snacks
		SUNDAY	
Cal.	Cal.	Cal.	Cal.

Weekend To-do's

List the types of exercises you will do this week and place an x on the day you plan to do them.

Exercise	Mon	Tue	Wed	Thur	Fri	Sat	Sun

Weekly Grocery List Sheets

Week # _____   _____ to _____ Total Spent $_____

Whole Grains	Produce

Dairy	Meat/Poultry/Fish/Deli

Condiments	Frozen

Canned Goods	Packaged Goods

Cleaning/Paper Supplies	Miscellaneous

Avoid:	Include:
Saturated fats	Good fats (olive oil, avocado, etc.)
Trans fats (partially hydrogenated oils)	Low-fat dairy and meats
Palm kernel oil, lard, shortening	High-fiber cereals (min. 5 grams)
Refined grains	100% whole-grain bread
Artificial flavorings	100% fruit juice
Olestra	Foods with no preservatives
Nitrates	Low-sodium canned goods
Hidden added sugars	Flavored green tea
Pastries, sodas, and sugary cereals	Raw nuts
Hidden sodium	Legumes
Full-fat meats	Beans and peas
Full-fat dairy	Deep-colored fruits and veggies

Daily Journal Sheets

Week #_____   _____ **to** _____

List everything you eat and drink each day. Be sure to track calories and food group servings too.

Breakfast	Lunch	Dinner	Snacks	Other
		MONDAY		Grain _____ Fruit _____ Veg _____ Meat _____ Dairy _____
Cal.	Cal.	Cal.	Cal.	Tot. Cal.

Breakfast	Lunch	Dinner	Snacks	Other
		TUESDAY		Grain _____ Fruit _____ Veg _____ Meat _____ Dairy _____
Cal.	Cal.	Cal.	Cal.	Tot. Cal.

Breakfast	Lunch	Dinner	Snacks	Other
				Grain _____
				Fruit _____
				Veg _____
				Meat _____
		WEDNESDAY		**Dairy** _____
Cal.	Cal.	Cal.	Cal.	Tot. Cal.

Breakfast	Lunch	Dinner	Snacks	Other
				Grain _____
				Fruit _____
				Veg _____
				Meat _____
		THURSDAY		**Dairy** _____
Cal.	Cal.	Cal.	Cal.	Tot. Cal.

Breakfast	Lunch	Dinner	Snacks	Other
				Grain _____
				Fruit _____
				Veg _____
				Meat _____
		FRIDAY		Dairy _____
Cal.	Cal.	Cal.	Cal.	Tot. Cal.

Breakfast	Lunch	Dinner	Snacks	Other
				Grain _____
				Fruit _____
				Veg _____
				Meat _____
		SATURDAY		Dairy _____
Cal.	Cal.	Cal.	Cal.	Tot. Cal.

Breakfast	Lunch	Dinner	Snacks	Other
				Grain _____
				Fruit _____
				Veg _____
		SUNDAY		Meat _____
				Dairy _____
Cal.	Cal.	Cal.	Cal.	Tot. Cal.

Exercise	Day of Week	Hrs/Min.	Calories Burned

Weekly Progress Report   Goal   Actual

Total calories consumed this week   _____   _____
Total calories burned this week   _____   _____
Total weight lost this week   _____   _____

Things I'll do next week to improve: _____

_____

_____

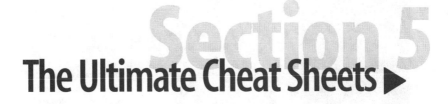

The Ultimate Cheat Sheets ▶

Contributors to Nutritional Bankruptcy

This cheat sheet outlines the leading food categories that contribute to obesity and the onset of chronic diseases. We suggest you try to limit these foods to no more than 10% of your overall daily diet. Check out our list of **"healthy substitutes"** on **Cheat Sheet #6** for great suggestions on how to replace some of the foods below with more healthy and tasty choices!

Food Type	Why They're Unhealthy	Examples
sugary beverages	high in calories, refined sugar, and artificial dyes	sodas, punches, and fruit drinks
processed grains	the good nutrients have been processed out, most of the important fiber, antioxidants, and minerals are lost	many breakfast cereals, some breads, white rice, pastries, and donuts
full-fat meats	high in saturated fats, calories, and some contain nitrates	prime rib, sausage, bacon, deli meats, hot dogs, and poultry with the skin
full-fat dairy	high in saturated fats and calories	"whole" milk, yogurt cheese, cream cheese, sour cream, and ice cream
unhealthy oils	hydrogenated; partially hydrogenated oils and saturated fats	lard, palm oil, coconut, oil , margarine, and vegetable shortening
fast foods	high in saturated fats, trans fats, and calories	double cheeseburgers, burgers with sauce, French fries, and hot dogs
commercially baked	high in processd white flour, trans fats, and refined sugar	donuts, pastries, pies, and cakes
packaged snacks	many contain trans fats, olestra, artificial ingredients, high sodium, and added sugars	many potato chips, crackers, cookies, and breakfast foods

Tips on Reading the "Front Label"

There are three areas on a packaged food item that you should get familiar with to keep your body healthy and slim. They include the "front label," the "ingredients list", and the "Nutrition Facts" label. Taken together, the information on all three labels will help you make the healthiest food choices possible. On the following pages, we give you tips on how to be a nutritionally savvy shopper. Referring to these cheat sheets when shopping for groceries can be a lifesaver!

Front Label Trickery

Manufacturers use the front label to entice shoppers to buy their products—it's pure advertising. Be aware of these "red flag" words found on the front label of many products.

Red Flags	What They Mean	Look For
fortified, enriched, added, extra, plus	the food has been processed in some way	no preservatives or made from 100% natural ingredients
fruit drinks	contains little fruit and a lot of sugar	100% fruit juice or no added sugar
wheat flour multi-grain	contains some whole wheat, but not much	whole grain 100% Whole Wheat
natural	started as a natural source but may end up anything but natural	100% all natural no preservatives
organically grown pesticide-free	may not be 100% organic	certified organically grown
sugar-free	might contain sugar alcohol which has as many calories as table sugar	sugarless or no added sugar

Tips on Reading the "Ingredients List"

The "ingredients list" label will help you find the hidden trans fats, sugars, sodium, artificial flavorings, and refined grains. In order to make it really simple, we've categorized these evildoer ingredients and listed the most common forms of each so that you can easily recognize them.

Evildoer Ingredients	Code Words
trans fats ▶	hydrogenated, partially hydrogenated oils
added sugar ▶	dextrose, lactose, sucrose, levulose, fructose, maltose, malt, corn syrup, maple sugar, raw sugar, brown sugar, glucose, turbinado, granulated sugar, mannitol, molasses, milk sugar, high fructose corn syrup, sorbitol, honey, xylitol, invert sugar, fruit juice concentrate, evaporated cane juice, and maltitol
added sodium ▶	baking soda, brine, disodium phosphate, garlic salt, onion salt, monosodium glutamate (MSG), salt, sodium alginate, sodium benzoate, sodium caseinate, sodium hydroxide, sodium nitrate, sodium pectinate, sodium proprionate, sodium sulfite, and soy sauce
refined grain ▶	enriched flour, wheat flour, or unbleached wheat flour
artificial color ▶	D&C Blue No. 1 & 2, FD&C Green No. 3, FD&C Red No. 1 & 40, and FD&C Yellow No. 5 & 6
miscellaneous ▶	olestra (fake fat), nitrates (found in cured meats)

Tips on Reading the "Nutrition Facts" Label

This label tells you the calories, total fat, saturated fat, cholesterol, sodium, total carbs (fiber and sugar,)and protein <u>in one serving from the food item</u>.Always check the number of servings per container. If you eat the whole package, multiply all of the nutritional information— including the calories—by this number. Below are a few tips on how to distinguish the nutrient content on the Nutrition Facts label:

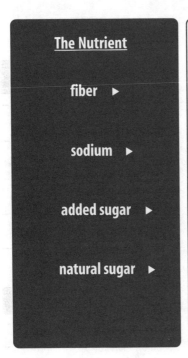

<u>The Nutrient</u>	<u>The Amount</u>(good/bad or high/low)
fiber ▶	2-3 grams is a good source 5 grams or more is considered high 10 grams or more is an excellent source
sodium ▶	35 grams is very low 140 grams is still low 400 grams is very high
added sugar ▶	5 grams or less is low over 15 grams is high 25 grams is extremely high
natural sugar ▶	any amount is acceptable for the following foods as long as there is no added sugar: milk, plain yogurt, fruit or veggie juice, fruits, and veggies

▶

Portion Control Tips

The secret to good health and weight management is making wise food choices and portion control, and this means adhering to the "standard" serving sizes of the various food groups. <u>**Below we provide approximate calorie counts**</u> (calories may differ slightly from brand to brand) to help you stay on track with your calorie budget! Consider this cheat sheet a calorie counter, measuring cup, and a food scale- all in one!

Whole Grains (Carbs)	**Serving Size**	**Eyeball**	**Calories**
Bread	1 slice	Large Palm	80
Bagel	½ of a small	½ palm	80
Pita	½ of regular	Large palm	80
Corn tortilla	1 (6")	Whole hand	80
Bran cereal	½ cup	Handful (cupped)	80
Dry cereal	½ cup	Handful (cupped)	100
Oatmeal	½ cup	Handful (cupped)	80
Rice	½ cup	Handful (cupped)	80
Pasta	½ cup	Handful (cupped)	80

Fruits (Carbs)	**Serving Size**	**Eyeball**	**Calories**
Whole small	1 piece	Fist	60
Raw chopped	½ cup	Handful (cupped)	60
Dried	3 oz	Handful (cupped)	200
Canned (no syrup)	½ cup	Handful (cupped)	60
Juice (unsweetened)	6 oz	Small juice cup	90

Veggies (Carbs)	**Serving Size**	**Eyeball**	**Calories**
Raw/chopped	½ cup	Handful (cupped)	25
Cooked	½ cup	Handful	25
Raw leafy	1 cup	Fist	25

Meat Group (Protein)	Serving Size	Eyeball	Calories
Lean beef/pork	3 oz	Palm	165
Lean poultry	3 oz	Palm	165
Fish	3 oz	Palm	165
Whole eggs	1 egg	Actual	75
Egg whites	¼ cup	Small handful	35
Beans/peas	½ cup	Handful	100
Peanut butter	2 T	2 thumb tips	200
Nuts (raw)	¼ cup	Small handful	200

Dairy/Alternative	Serving Size	Eyeball	Calories
Skim milk	1 cup	Fist	90
Low-fat milk (1%)	1 cup	Fist	110
Milk (2%)	1 cup	Fist	120
Enriched soy milk	1 cup	Fist	100
Yogurt, plain, non-fat	1 cup	Fist	130
Yogurt, fruit, low-fat	1 cup	Fist	150
Low-fat natural cheese	1 ounce	Thumb	80

Fats	Serving Size	Eyeball	Calories
Most oils	1 T	1 Thumb	120
Most nuts	¼ cup	Small handful	200
Avocados	1 T	1 Thumb	120

Healthy Substitutes for Common Foods

In keeping with our mode of simplicity, we created this cheat sheet for you to use as a great reference tool when planning your weekly meals and creating your grocery lists. We've taken some of the most common foods and found healthier substitutes for you to choose from. Once you start incorporating these healthier choices into your diet, you'll find that you don't have to give up great taste to eat healthier! The healthy substitutes listed below are better choices because they include one or more of the following:

Fewer calories   **Less fat**
No trans fats   **Less added sugar**
More fiber   **More antioxidants**

These food selections are based on the standard serving size for each food listed.

Popular Food	The Makeover	The Payoff
spaghetti	whole wheat	adds 3g of fiber
sugary cereal	high-fiber cereal	adds 12g of fiber
multi-grain bread	100% whole wheat	adds 2g of fiber
flour tortillas	corn tortillas	saves 45 calories
white rice	brown rice	adds 1g of fiber and B vitamins
regular tortilla chips	organic blue chips	no trans fat, adds 2g of fiber
regular peanut butter	all natural peanut butter	no trans fats
regular ground beef	extra lean ground beef	saves 12g of fat and 100 calories
pork chop	pork tenderloin	saves 5g of fat and 45 calories

Popular Food	The Makeover	The Payoff
deli sliced ham	deli sliced turkey breast	saves 3g of fat and 60 calories, contains no nitrates
flavored yogurt	plain yogurt	saves 15g of sugar
2% milk	skim milk	saves 5g of fat and 40 calories
cheddar cheese	low-fat cheddar cheese	saves 3g fat and 65 calories
Swiss cheese	low-fat Swiss cheese	saves 4g of fat and 50 calories
regular ice cream	low-fat frozen yogurt	saves 11g of fat and 120 calories
cream cheese	low-fat cream cheese	saves 5g of fat and 25 calories
cottage cheese	low-fat cottage cheese	saves 4g of fat and 35 calories
regular mayo	low-fat mayo	saves 6g of fat and 50 calories
sour cream	low-fat sour cream	saves 5g of fat and 40 calories
salad dressing	low-cal dressing	saves 10g of fat and 50 calories
butter	olive oil	no trans fats
iced tea	green tea	adds antioxidants

Dining Out Without Pigging Out

Restaurants and fast food places serve portions that are two to five times larger than they were in the 1950's. So, it's more important than ever to use all your "hand tricks" to estimate standard serving sizes, as well as these helpful hints below.

Fast Food Tips

Burgers
Order the smallest possible size. Try to hold off on the cheese, bacon, mayo, and creamy sauces. Instead, opt for mustard, ketchup, and fresh veggies.

Chicken
Be aware that deep-fried chicken, coated chicken, and chicken nuggets are extremely high in fat and calories. Flame-grilled chicken is a good choice, but be sure to remove the skin. Chicken sandwiches and pitas are good choices, as long as they are grilled and served without the creamy, fat-laden sauces.

Fish
The same tips that apply to choosing a healthy chicken meal, apply to fish meals. Choose grilled fish and forgo the creamy, fat-laden sauces.

Fries
Instead of fries or onion rings, try a plain baked potato with reduced-fat dressing or choose a side salad with low-fat dressing. Carrot and raisin salad is another great alternative. If you absolutely must have fries, order the small and split them with someone, or throw half of them out!

Pizza
Good news, this can actually be a very healthy meal—if you follow these tips. Always choose the thin crust, add as many vegetable toppings as possible, and avoid the salami, pepperoni, bacon, mince, and the tempting extra cheese option. In fact, you can request less cheese and no one will know the difference!

Restaurant Tips

Since restaurants offer so many tempting selections, the last thing you want to do is arrive starving! We recommend that you have a healthy snack just before you go to curb your hunger. Also, try to decide in advance what you will eat and be sure to follow the tips below—you'll have a better chance of staying within your daily calorie budget.

◄ Many restaurants offer half portions of their meals as well as a lite and healthy menu, be sure to ask.

◄ Be creative with the menu. Take advantage of healthy appetizers and order these as your main entrée, the serving size is more in line with your new eating plan.

◄ Another great way to keep portions in line is to split your dinner with someone else. Or if no one wants to split, have the waiter put half of the meal in a to-go box **before** you are served.

◄ Keep extras like the bread, desserts, regular sodas, sweetened tea, and alcoholic beverages to a minimum. Everything counts!!

◄ Order grilled fish whenever possible for the health benefits (salmon and tuna are the best).

◄ Ask to have your dinner prepared with light oil. The kitchen is usually happy to comply.

◄ Order things "Meg Ryan" style with either the fattening stuff "on the side" or delete it altogether—like full-fat cheeses, salad dressings, extra butter, and creamy sauces.

◄ Order your food baked, steamed, or grilled, **NOT** fried!

◄ Fill your plate up with fruits, veggies, and salads to ensure that you are meeting your 5-10 daily quota! **Note:** Make sure they are not doused in creamy sauces or butter.

◄ For dessert go for fresh berries, fruit salad, or flavored tea.

◄ Stick to wine or beer rather than high-cal, high-sugar drinks like Pina Coladas and Margaritas.

◄ Be sure to drink plenty of water, this will give you something to do with your hands and make you feel fuller, which will help you stick to your plan.

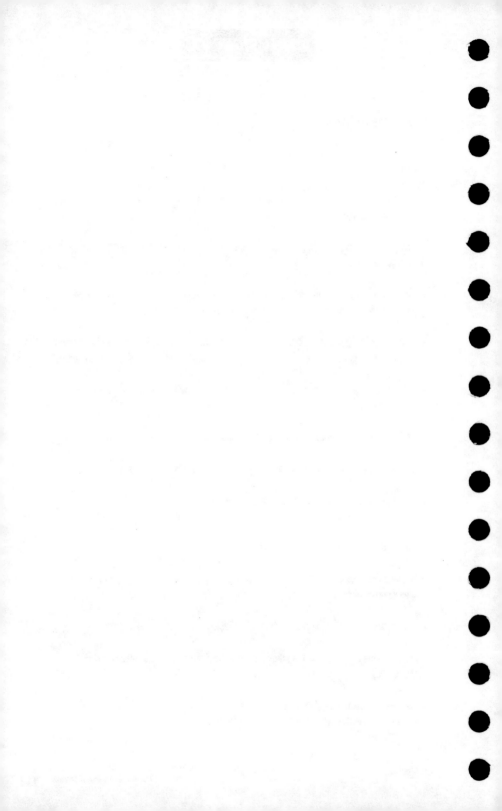

About the Author

Kerry McLeod is a graduate of the University of Texas, with a B.S. in Psychology. She spent the first 15 years of her career working for Fortune 500 companies such as Cox Enterprises, Inc., and McGraw-Hill Publishing in various sales and marketing positions. In 2001, nine months after the birth of her daughter, she left the safe world of the corporate "gravy train" and cautiously entered the challenging and oftentimes treacherous world of the stay-at-home/working-from-home moms' club. Currently, she is a freelance marketing consultant, Sports Nutrition Certified Instructor, and a full-time wife and mother.

Kerry also has the title of "recovering junk-food junkie" on her resume. For most of her adult life, her diet consisted of empty calories from highly processed foods, sans anything remotely healthy. In her early thirties, she decided it was time to change her evil diet and nutrition ways and began looking for an easy-to-implement eating plan that she could apply to the real world—hers. Over the next seven years, she tried many diet plans, but found that they were either too complicated, too labor-intensive, or too restrictive—no dairy, no mixing carbs and proteins, low carb, high protein, and of course the dreaded no sugar! Although she was eating better, she still hadn't found a healthy plan that she could follow for life, and so the search continued.

Then one day several years ago, she had her light-bulb moment: If she was having this much trouble figuring out the whole nutrition and weight loss game, then what were other women going through who weren't as informed as she? This is when she decided there was a real need for a no-nonsense, simple nutrition and weight loss program that could be applied to any lifestyle. With this, she set out to create the ultimate eating plan for women! And the rest, as they say, is history.

www.simplenutritionseries.com

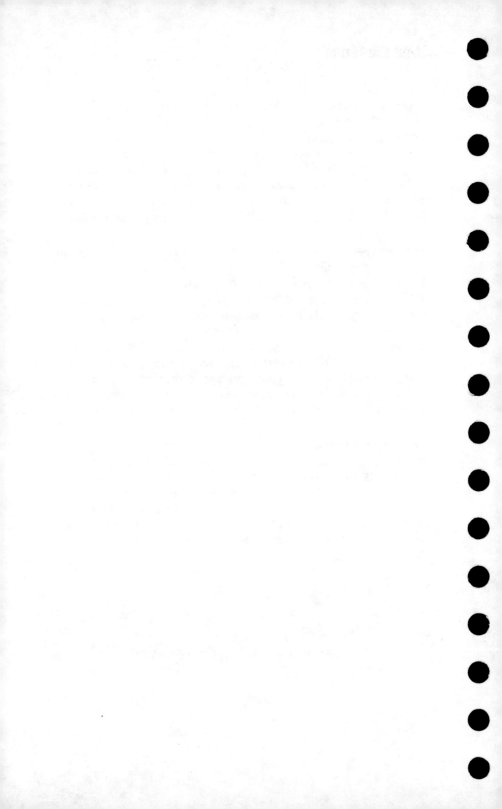